The Miracle of Hospice

Mary,

Blessings to you always and thank you for all that you bring to our hospice team. May you be filled with Love + Light

Cathy True

The Miracle of Hospice

A Personal Journey of a Hospice Nurse

Cathy Truehart

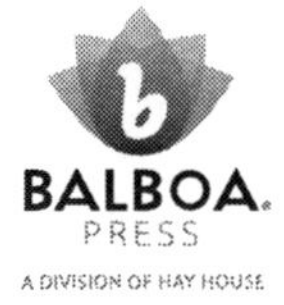

ISBN: 978-1-4525-5083-1 (sc)
ISBN: 978-1-4525-5082-4 (e)

Balboa Press books may be ordered through booksellers or by contacting:

Balboa Press
A Division of Hay House
1663 Liberty Drive
Bloomington, IN 47403
www.balboapress.com
1-(877) 407-4847

Because of the dynamic nature of the Internet, any web addresses or links contained in this book may have changed since publication and may no longer be valid. The views expressed in this work are solely those of the author and do not necessarily reflect the views of the publisher, and the publisher hereby disclaims any responsibility for them.

The author of this book does not dispense medical advice or prescribe the use of any technique as a form of treatment for physical, emotional, or medical problems without the advice of a physician, either directly or indirectly. The intent of the author is only to offer information of a general nature to help you in your quest for emotional and spiritual well-being. In the event you use any of the information in this book for yourself, which is your constitutional right, the author and the publisher assume no responsibility for your actions.

Printed in the United States of America

Balboa Press rev. date:8/29/2012

Dedication

This book is dedicated to the hospice patients
it has been my privilege to serve,
and from whom I have received so much,

and to my devoted husband Richard Truehart,
with all gratitude and love.

Contents

To The Reader

This is an unabashedly personal account of my education as a hospice nurse and the experiences of some of those I have been privileged to serve. I hope to help people alleviate, or at least balance, the dread or even panic so many patients and family members experience when they first hear the word "hospice." By writing personally and in detail about the day-to-day process of hospice and hospice nursing, I hope to dispel some of the stigma the very word produces.

It is my intention to let my heart speak through my words. Rather than try to duplicate the many excellent materials that are available to explain terminal illness, pain management, hospice and other such issues from an objective or clinical viewpoint, I simply want to provide one woman's perspective on her day to day journeys among them. I emphasize that the material in this book represents my personal opinion, and I encourage all of you who are interested in doing so to explore other hospice resources further. Also, please note that names and case details have been changed to protect the privacy of the patients and families whose stories are shared herein.

As you will quickly see, the theme of this book is not just death and dying, but also life and hope. The principles of hospice were designed specifically to provide the seriously ill with help that focuses on the quality of their lives, rather than a rush toward any and all possible "cures" no matter how painful or unlikely. In part because of this focus on their comfort and well-being, patients are actually discharged from hospices all over the world far more often that most lay persons imagine. There is no such thing as "no hope"; as this book suggests, miracles—of all kinds—do happen.

Introduction

My first official work with hospice began in the late 70s, while I was going to school for my B.S.N. in Public Health Nursing in Cotati, California. The first time I heard the word hospice and learned what it meant, I somehow knew that this would become my life's work.

But my passion for the exploration of death and dying actually started at the age of five in a lake in Maine. Called Porter Lake, it was located in New Vineyard, a town whose population could not have been more than 500 or so. It was there that I had the near-death experience that, symbolically enough, began my life's work.

I was swimming in the lake with my mother, my sister, and a few friends. The lake itself was muddy and infested with leeches, which we would have to peel off our skin when we emerged from the water. Inner tube around my waist, I was practicing my diving skills. You can probably guess where this story is going already. The older children were diving off the larger rocks with my sister, while I was restricted to the big flat rock that skimmed the surface of the water. My mother made the mistake of telling me that I was doing so well that I would soon be diving as well as my sister. With newfound confidence, I decided to "crank up" my diving a notch. I dove into the water head first, with my inner tube securely around my waist. Once under the water, though, it held me securely pinned there.

As almost everyone who undergoes a near death experience reports, I recall each and every detail as though it happened yesterday. I believe this was the first time I had ever opened my eyes under water, and I remember being amazed to see beautiful, tropically colorful fish swimming above the clear sandy bottom. In reality, the water was as black as a boot, and probably inhabited only by algae and the creatures we called "blood suckers." I saw my mother's legs through the water. She was standing nearby, "counting heads" and making sure all of the children were safe. Knowing that my ever-loving, always trustworthy mother was close by my side made me feel even more secure.

I vividly recall my amazement at my ability to breathe under water. I had always been taught that this was impossible but by golly, here I was, breathing with ease. I was full of wonder, curiosity, and peace.

Then, "let there be light!" I remember a beautiful white light illuminating the lake. It was a magical glow. I no longer felt as though I was in water; instead, I somehow experienced myself as part of the lovely light. I saw nothing and heard nothing, just felt a sense of peace, calm, and beauty.

Unbeknownst to me, my mother had seen my legs flailing wildly and frantically. She told me later that she could clearly see me "fighting for my life." She got me pulled out of the water. I was gasping and choking, but my breath normalized without the requirement of artificial resuscitation. My mother was of course terrified. There had been a record number of drownings at the pond that year.

Much later, I came across a book explaining that drowning was one of the most beautiful ways to die. I don't remember now who wrote this or how they knew, but I felt that I could attest to the truth of the words. I have since spoken to others who had near-death drowning experiences like mine, but did not have a wondrous or positive experience.

To this day, the vision I had of the passage between life and death remains one of my most treasured experiences. From that moment on, my life took on a new meaning and focus. Unlike most people, I have never feared death. To the contrary, I knew that it was an amazing experience: something I could contemplate with wonder, awe, and trust.

I want to emphasize that my thoughts on death were not a "morbid" preoccupation. I didn't brood on death or dying, or look forward to it happening to me any time soon. I took for granted that I would live a long, rich life. The clearest way to explain my feelings might be just to say that for me, death had become a part of life, one of the many amazing experiences it offered, something to revere rather than fear. That day at the lake, I had come to see death as holy and natural rather than scary.

Naturally, even as a child I wanted to share my newfound confidence and reverence with others. When I had to choose a topic for classroom presentations, I would select death or dying. I'm sure that many of my listeners, both adults and children, felt that this was odd. But it seemed totally normal to me.

And so, it is no coincidence that I am a hospice nurse today. People often ask, "How can you do this work? Isn't it depressing?" The answer, for me, is "no." I can honestly tell them that it is my life's work, my passion, my ministry. I find joy and comfort in ministering to those on this sacred journey, and I hope I offer comfort as well.

Where appropriate, I share my experience with my patients and their families in hopes that it will help alleviate their fear or dread. I also share my memory of being peaceful and amazed by the closeness of death, even at a time when my mother saw me struggling against it. I hope that they are able to take comfort in the peaceful transition described by someone who has undergone it at least part of the way, and in the assurance that a loved one who is manifesting the physical symptoms of approaching death—and even appear to be struggling—may actually be in the kind of peaceful, beautiful place that I experienced deep in the lake.

For me, hospice is a profoundly spiritual journey. Preparing, supporting, and being a witness to those who are crossing over to the other side seems to me like the closest you can get to God and the spirit world. It is not a burden but a privilege to be able to accompany people on part of this sacred journey. It is my hope that through this book I can share with you some of this sense of privilege and wonder. In my story, I hope you can see first hand how I and so many others can not only do this sometimes challenging work, but love doing so as well.

Part One: One Day

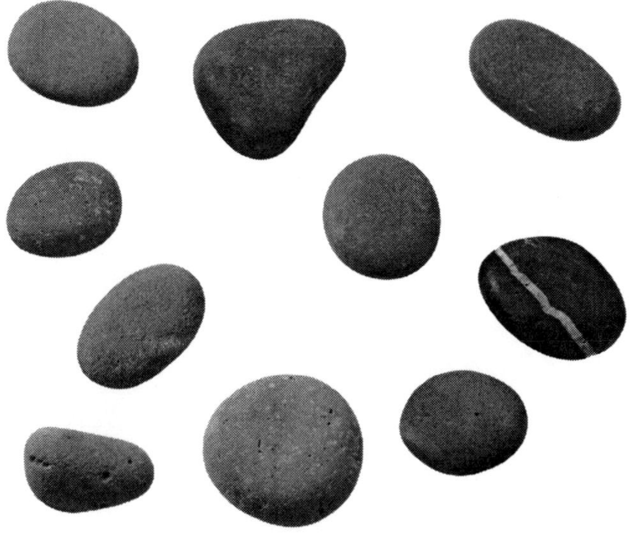

Death is not the enemy to be conquered or a prison to be escaped.
It is an integral part of our lives that gives meaning to human experience. It sets a limit on our time in this life, urging us on to do something productive with that time as long as it is ours to use.
—Joseph and Laurie Braga, Foreword *to Elisabeth Kübler-Ross's* Death, The Final Stage of Growth

The Day Begins

Have you ever had a day when you felt as though you were in a movie *and* you had the leading role…and not in the glamorous sense? For me, the single twenty-four-hour span I share in this section was exactly that kind of day.

The actual tasks that hospice nurses perform are incredibly varied, and that May weekday illustrated their diversity to an almost comical degree. I went from performing medical tasks like catheterizations to cleaning kitty litter boxes…from having a personal epiphany on a porch to sitting on a patient's bed hearing precious life stories…from doing a pronouncement of death to breaking up a fistfight in a family meeting… all ending with a visit to a patient who had actually been discharged from our service. The saying "all in a day's work" seemed all too true that day. When it was finally done I thought, "I could write a book about this day!" At the time I meant that it was quite an experience, but here I am eight years later, and it still seems like the perfect day to use as an example of all the many paradoxes of hospice and hospice care. One of the cases mentioned happened at an earlier date.

When I am able to make time, I like to start my day with a morning meditation. Days that begin with this silent and centering time always seem to go much more smoothly than the days when I rush straight into the tasks of everyday life. Thanks to my husband, who built our home, I have a small room set aside just for this purpose. It is filled with holy objects that have special meaning to me. These include pictures and statues of Christ, a large Brazilian amethyst crystal geode, a statue of the Buddha, Native American artifacts, and a beautiful tree stump. As you can immediately tell, my spirituality does not fit into any one religious denomination; as I'll explain in more detail later in this book, I respect, and draw strength, from many different traditions. In addition, rocks and stones are everywhere, in that little room and in our house. I gather them from the beaches and lakesides I visit. I love their subtle colors and shapes. For me, they speak of the history of the earth, its information and strength, its endurance. I feel a kinship with them, and for me they seem to have a life all their own.

On this day, I settled myself among these precious objects and began my mediation practice. Soon the face of my patient Roger came to my mind. I paid attention to this "visit," as things like this are often helpful intuitive tips on how the day will go. I was reminded that Roger had told me that this was the day he was going to die. I trust everything a dying person tells me as they are virtually always right.

So I had listened carefully to Roger's assessment of his own situation. Thanks to his "visit" in my meditation session, I felt guided to bring the new sage stick I had purchased after my first visit with him. Used widely in Native American tradition, sage is a sacred herb that is burned to purify the air and cleanse the body. Roger and I had never spoken of this tradition, yet I felt some kind of deeper "knowing" that this was exactly what he would want. Situations like this always remind me of what a relatively small role words play in communication. Studies suggest that only seven percent of communication is verbal, while the other 93 percent is nonverbal. I'm not a statistician, but my personal experience suggests that those proportions are pretty accurate. Roger will be discussed more fully later "in the day."

I finished my meditation and gathered my things, including the sage stick. It was a beautiful, sunny day, the kind those of us who live in the Northeast welcome after the long winter. I got into my 1987 red Sebring convertible and put the top down so that I could enjoy the air and sunshine. My drives to, from and between appointments are very important to me. Even on days when the trip is filled with ice, sleet or snow rather than sunshine, they give me a chance to regroup in between each new case or task. Because I tend to absorb the energy around me like a sponge, these periodic chances to ground myself are crucial to me. In truth, I am not sure I could do hospice nursing in a single, enclosed setting.

Before I started my drive I put a Carolyn Myss tape in the player and pushed start. Carolyn Myss is my favorite spiritual "mentor." I listen to her material over and over again, and learn something new each time. Each hearing inspires me anew. Today, appropriately, I was listening to her book *The Science of Medical Intuition*. Her wise words, combined with the sunshine and my beloved car, were an energizing start to the day.

Mr. & Mrs. L.

As often happens in my work, today I got re-routed from the appointment I expected to make in response to a patient call. Mr. L—neither he nor his wife were informal, first-name people—had prostate cancer. The call told me he had a blocked Foley catheter, and I received it with some apprehension, unsure I would be able to reinsert the blocked catheter smoothly. I also felt awkward about having spent time talking to Mrs. L about her beautiful homemade quilts, rather than getting to the task at hand. I usually trust that such things will play out as per a divine plan in the end, but that doesn't mean that doubts don't creep in at times. As it happened, I was able to fix the problem without difficulty. I phoned the doctor in charge to receive medication orders and had the chance to speak "heart to heart" with Mrs. L.

She wanted to speak about the timeframe of her husband's journey. I told her that I thought this might be his last weekend. She replied that she had suspected as much, but she was grateful for the confirmation so that she could gather friends and family. I left the house glad that the catheter problem had brought me there, and given me the opportunity to support not only Mr. L himself but also his wife.

Lina

My next destination was only a few streets away. Lina was an eight-year-old girl who had been diagnosed with a brain tumor at the age of only two and a half. The cancer had metastasized to her spinal cord. As a result, she had been paralyzed from the neck down for the past two months. I had admitted her to our hospice service ten months before, at which time the doctors had estimated that she had only a few months to live.

Lina had been through many surgeries by this time—there had been nine in all, I believe. One surgery had caused one of her eyes to cross, while the high doses of steroids she was on to shrink the tumors made her little cheeks puffy and her belly swollen and firm. Her mouth was somewhat crooked, pushing toward the left side in the same way the mouth of someone who had had a stroke might look. She was about three and a half feet tall, but the severity of her physical challenges meant that I rarely saw her standing up. Despite these many challenges, she remained in many ways a perfectly normal little girl. Like so many children her age, she was obsessed with Barney, the purple dinosaur from T.V. He had a special place among the many stuffed animals piled on the bed where she spent almost all of her time.

Lina had thick black shoulder-length hair. Brushing her hair was a special task that only her daddy Joe was allowed to do. In fact, her father was the only person she wanted to handle all aspects of her daily care. Only he could bathe, feed, medicate, move, and (late in her illness, when she could no longer walk to the bathroom) change her. Certainly, this was no reflection on her mother Liz, a schoolteacher. There was no doubt about Lina's love for her mother, her mother's love for her, or the quality of her mother's care. Lina was simply a "Daddy's girl" through and through.

In addition to taking a long leave of absence from his job, Joe limited his sleep to only a few hours a night, and even then slept "with one ear open" in case Lina needed him. He took such joy in the simple pleasures of touching his daughter's cheeks, brushing her hair, and propping her up in bed with all of her favorite "stuffies" around her. His eyes would gleam with pleasure and pride when he shared their special moments. For example, he told me that he loved to hear her little voice call "God bless you, Daddy" when he sneezed in the night. I think I remember him commenting that he sometimes faked a sneeze just to hear that. He loved to hear her sing along with all of her favorite T.V. shows and talk in her "teddy bear voice" as well.

When I first met Lina, her personality was different than I expected. Most of us (even those of us who are parents and should know better!) expect children to be sweet and docile. This was exactly what I expected from Lina before we met. I guess I pictured some sort of sentimental, "best buddies" situation like the ones you find in movies. WRONG! Lina might have been physically weak, but she was not emotionally passive in the least. She always called the shots, and she was bright and argumentative enough to get her way most of the time. Lina was notorious for dismissing people whom she did not like. She ordered these poor folks to leave, sparing no feelings.

Certainly, this approach could make her care challenging. Yet in some ways it was also very healthy. Adults struggling with serious illness often feel so dependent on, or burdensome to, others that they stop advocating strongly enough for what they want. Lina's sense that her emotions were important—that she had a right to define at least some of the parameters within which her care was given—almost certainly helped her survive.

Volunteers play a key role in hospice services. Many of them have had a personal experience with hospice during a family member's death, and wish to give back. It is no exaggeration to say that hospice work could not be done without these extraordinary people. One of our most special volunteers, Theresa, turned out to be a real favorite with Lina, second only to her father. Shallow as it sounds, I have to admit that I would ordinarily be jealous of Lina's obvious favorite. Hospice workers do not leave their human foibles behind when they come to work, and we all want to be valued by those we serve closely. But it was such a joy to see Lina come alive with Theresa, that my human foibles disappeared and I felt truly happy to witness the closeness between them.

Theresa worked with hand puppets, and brought a group of them with her on each of her twice-weekly visits. Lina would speak of her pain or illness only in third person, through the puppets' mouths. The rest of the time she refused to acknowledge pain, even when it was very visible on her little face or body. In the eleven months I worked with her, I never heard her complain a single time. Instead, she always insisted that nothing was wrong with her. Given that, Theresa and her puppets provided some very valuable information to Lina's parents and care team—information I don't believe could have been garnered in any more conventional way.

For the first few months of my care for Lina, we would sit and color together. Lina would scold me every time I failed to put a crayon back in its proper spot—which I inevitably did, because only Lina herself knew the rightful place of each color. Once Lina became bedridden, coloring was no longer an option. I felt anxious about what to do at each visit. Making things even more awkward, Liz, Lina's mom, had told her daughter that only very old or very sick people die. As I've previously noted, I am usually comfortable speaking about death. But I did not want to have to contradict Lina's mother in any way when speaking to her child. So I found myself avoiding any conversation on this subject. In the end, the only thing Lina ever said to me about death was to ask if she would have her hospital bed in heaven. Later, very shortly before her death, she asked me, "Why hasn't God come to get me?"

May 2nd became an important visit day with Lina and her Dad. During that visit, I did all the things I usually did at Lina's home. I checked on Lina first. Then, Joe and I reviewed her medications and their ever-changing dosages, so that I could make any necessary recommendations for adjustments. He was amazing at keeping this copious information straight. At the end of each visit, I would call Lina's two doctors. This isn't a customary part of hospice nursing, but both of these physicians were deeply attentive to this patient, and welcomed regular updates.

Once the medication had been reviewed, Joe and I sat together on the family's back porch. Lina was asleep, and sitting outside allowed us to spend a few quiet moments in the fresh, warm air. During such times together I got to know a lot about this courageous man and his family's situation. He shared memories of his siblings, of his meeting and courtship with Lina's mother, and other family situations. Over time, he also filled me in on the long medical journey his family had walked before I met them. I found his confidences touching, because Joe had a deep distrust for social workers and the other professionals who, he felt, pried into his life.

I'm not sure exactly what we were talking about that May 2nd on his porch. I only know that I had a kind of epiphany—the kind of insight that comes like the proverbial bolt out of the blue. I wasn't really, or at least entirely, there for Lina, I realized. It didn't really matter what she did or did not let me do. I was there for Joe, as his support, his confidante, his consultant and most importantly his friend. The same was true for Liz, Lina's mom, though our times together took a completely different direction. Liz and I cried a lot, and we hugged a lot. Joe would always dismiss himself from our company with a small joke about the two of us "cry babies." We would laugh a little, then get back to our business of crying, hugging, talking about angels, or just complaining teasingly about men. It didn't matter what we said; what mattered was the togetherness, the warmth, and the sense of closeness and support.

My visits to Lina's family and all my other patients became so much easier that day. I no longer felt the old anxiety of "what do I do now?" or "is this right?" From that time on, I began to trust that my presence was as important as my actions. It also made me aware that I am there for family and friends as much as for the patient. Time with them is not time off from our work, but part of our work itself. This realization felt important and healing to me—a holy episode of the kind most of us experience only rarely.

That day also reminded me how much I myself gained from these times with a patient or family. As heart-wrenching as Lina's case was, words can't express what an honor it was to be a part of this family team for eleven months. What a privilege it was to witness this father devoting his entire life to the nurturing of his daughter, to share in this mother's grief, and to witness the courage and strength of this child they loved so much. For all of us as hospice providers, it is important to work within our policies and guidelines and to maintain appropriate boundaries with our clients. Yet at a deeper level, it is also true that we are all equal in the face of death and dying. In some sense, there is no caregiver and patient, expert and non-expert on this sacred ground.

Naturally, on May 2nd, I could not know how much more time I would have with Lina and her family. I visited as often and as extensively as I could, staying for longer than it would have taken just to do the required tasks. Hospice work always reminds you how precious the present moment is, and how much it must be savored.

Lina died that August. I had a very special time with her shortly before her death. Joe had gone out for a quick errand and Liz, with whom I had been sitting and crying in Lina's room, had left the room to take a phone call. Lina was unresponsive that day. She did not blink, or follow my fingers with her eyes. I can't explain precisely why but I felt guided to take the chance to give her the gentle hug and kiss she had never allowed.

I told her how much I loved her, and reassured her that it was okay to go into the light. I spoke of what a beautiful place she was going to, how she could bring all of her teddies there, and how there was nothing to be afraid of. I explained that her father, mother and brother would be okay, and that though her body would not be with them, her spirit would be here forever. I told her how important her life had been to so many people and how much joy she had brought her family, especially her daddy. I concluded by telling her that she was the strongest and bravest little girl I had ever met. Most of these things had probably been said to her many times by then, yet it felt important to me to speak the words myself as well.

I got no response from Lina, but I knew that I had done what I needed to. Joe came home then, and walked into her room. The moment he spoke, she snapped out of her semi-coma and began to speak to him. There was never any mention of my words to her, and that felt fine to me.

I was called to the family's house to make the pronouncement of death on the August day she died. Lina had died just the way she lived: strong-willed and in control, arguing every inch of the way. But her very end was peaceful, a gift for which I (and no doubt many others) had been praying for. When I arrived at the house, I found both of her doctors already there—a true "first" in all of my experience. The house was full of those who loved her, including her psychologist and her minister. The family insisted on waiting for Theresa, Lina's beloved Hospice volunteer, to arrive before any further arrangements were completed. Theresa was on vacation two hours away, but she was able to fulfill her deep desire to be there. When she arrived, she performed her final puppet show for Lina. It was obvious how deeply everyone in the house that day loved this little girl, and how privileged we all felt at being there together after her passing.

I would not have missed Lina's wake, funeral or memorial service for the world, so my family changed its vacation plans so that I could attend. I usually try to go to services for my patients for the families' sakes, but this time I was there as much for me as for them. Rather than being there "for" the family, this time I truly felt that I *was* family. Liz, Lina's mom, had once sent me a card that read, "When I see you, I don't see a nurse, I see a wonderful friend." It felt exactly the same to me. This family, and Lina herself, will live in my heart for eternity.

- There has never been a wake or funeral that has touched me as deeply as this one. The services were beautiful, tender, and lovingly personal. There were balloons and flowers everywhere, in the shape of Barney, Cinderella and all of her favorite characters. A video about Lina played; beautifully

> done and healing, it celebrated her life rather than focusing on her passing. At the funeral, Lina's brother, Juan, sang and recited a piece he had written called *The Twelve Gifts of Lina*. Lina had adored him, and he her. Seven years older than she was, Juan had coped well, both with her illness and with the way she was necessarily the center of attention—both difficult changes for a sibling. Watching him play this special role at her funeral was moving for all of us in attendance—and, I hope, healing for him as well.

Butterflies were released at the grave side where Lina was buried. One landed, ever so deliberately, on Liz's shoulder. It stayed for a while—a *long* while: a "coincidence" that felt just right, and one of my many special memories of that day.

Carolyn

By the time I finished at Lina's, it was noon. My schedule for the day was running very late, as I had only seen two people in four hours. The shepherd's pie I had eaten for breakfast having long since given way to hunger pangs, I ate a Pink Lady apple in the car. The food and the bright, sunny day I was driving through in my convertible felt heavenly and nurturing. I arrived at the house of my next patient restored, and with the same enthusiasm I would feel going to visit my dearest friend in the world.

Carolyn was a seventy-eight year old woman at that time. Widowed and with no children, she had been diagnosed with liver cancer seven months before. Her only living relations were a brother who lived out of state, and a nephew with health problems, whom I had only met once. Unlike Lina's home, which was filled with caregivers, Carolyn dealt with her final illness mostly alone.

Carolyn and I were definitely kindred spirits—two peas in a pod, you might say. We recognized this in the other and enjoyed our special bond. One sign of this special relationship was the way Carolyn left the door unlocked for me so that I could get in whenever I arrived. As a hospice nurse I am almost always racing the clock—and the clock always seems to win. I no sooner tell someone the time I will be at their door than some emergency arises or a conversation becomes too personal and too painful to cut short. I loved the fact that Carolyn was okay with my unpredictable schedule and also the way she just trusted that I would be there as soon as I could.

Despite the bright clear sunshine outside on this day, Carolyn and I sat where we always did, in her rather stuffy, cluttered living room, which was full of papers. Understandably, she did not have the energy to put them away or to wash the dishes that accumulated. As a hospice nurse, I don't have the time to take care of household chores. There are others charged with doing so and my schedule is just too crowded. Carolyn was the exception. We were close enough that I was glad to take on some of the extra tasks when I could. It seemed a minor gesture but it made a real difference in her situation once her health began to fail seriously and she could no longer walk with ease.

Carolyn loved television, and almost always had her T.V. set on. This May 2nd, I sat beside her, competing with the early-afternoon programs. Her cat, which was the center of her life, always joined us as well. He was a mangy creature with half of his hair missing, but he loved Carolyn and adored being petted. Carolyn often cracked jokes about which of them would die first, but she admitted in more serious moments that she was concerned about what would happen to him if she died before he did.

Fortunately, Carolyn did not have physical pain. But in addition to her growing problems with walking, she had a terrible rash all over her body. Caused by the disease in her liver, it was a never-ending agony that nothing we tried seemed to abate. She would often itch until she bled, creating welts and scabs on her body and bloodstains on her sheets. I rubbed her down with lotion, though it only gave her a few minutes of respite. I also took a minute to sit down on the bed afterward so that she would have a bit more company.

Today, she was reminiscing about her mother, who was an orphan, and her grandmother, who had practiced as a medium. She told me she still had the sign for her grandmother's psychic business. I was fascinated by this detail and wanted to dig the sign out of her attic, but as usual I had no time to do this now. Instead, I made her a snack, reordered the necessary medication, filled her pill box for the week, and cleaned the kitty litter box—one of my "special" tasks. That pretty much used up the time I had, so I gave her a hug and a kiss before racing off to a scheduled family meeting. It was located about thirty minutes from Carolyn's home, and I had just enough time to make it.

Jim

Some of the patients and families I serve as a hospice nurse come into my life only briefly and then disappear once my work with them ends. Others seem connected in more enduring ways. Jim, my next patient, was one of the latter.

I had first met Jim when I acted as the case manager for his brother, who had died on our hospice service about six months before. In his early seventies at that time, Jim had devoted the last years of his life caring for this brother, who had special needs. Then Jim himself had gotten lung cancer, which had now metastasized to the bone. As I drove toward his house, I reflected on my gratitude for being able to help care for him, just as he had cared for his brother.

Jim was a sweetheart, and I loved him dearly. He was soft-spoken, loyal, and giving. His family...well, as kids say today, not so much. It goes without saying that every family has its own complex dynamics, which illness or imminent death can exacerbate. Such was the case with Jim's family. I felt less like a nurse than a referee for a wrestling match when I was scheduled to facilitate a family meeting like the one planned for May 2nd.

Family conflicts don't sound like they have anything to do with a nurse's role, and in theory, that's true. In reality, however, the boundary around what our job is and what it isn't can't always be perfectly maintained. The messiness and the connectedness of human life often "bleed" through. This happened in Jim's case not only because I already knew his family, but also because managing family conflicts was integral to his comfort and care.

One night that past winter when I happened to be on call, for example, the wife of Jim's son Sam called me at around midnight, fit to be tied. Hot baths helped manage Jim's pain better than anything else, especially because he was resistant to pain medication. On that particular night, it seemed that Sam, who was something of a drinker, had gotten his father into the bathtub and then passed out. His wife, Jessica, could neither wake Sam up nor get Jim out of the tub and into bed by herself; in addition, she was understandably uncomfortable at the thought of moving her naked father-in-law around! He weighed less than one hundred pounds by this time, but that's a lot of weight when you are a small person trying to get someone else's wet, slippery, and fragile body safely moved.

It was a thirty-minute drive from my home to theirs. By the time I arrived, Jim was as shriveled-up as a prune. I got him out of the tub and I half-walked, half-carried him down two steps, then up another three, into his room. He paused at the landing and said, "You know, you're all right!" "You know, you're all right too, Jim," I said, smiling back.

That one moment made getting up at midnight a pleasure rather than a burden. It was the kind of tender, happy moment hospice can (paradoxically) give, and one I knew I'd always cherish. Another such exchange occurred later that winter, right after Sam and I had gotten his father clean and comfortable. Jim was bedridden and very weak at that time. Despite this, he had a twinkle in his eye when he looked up at me and said, "If I was twenty years younger, I'd jump up and give you a kiss!" Without a second thought I leaned over him and gave him that kiss. That clearly pleased Jim, and made Sam laugh as well—and as always, laughter is a healing release for everyone involved.

I don't remember exactly what had led to the family meeting that was held on May 2nd. Probably, Sam had been threatening to leave as a result of his latest conflict with Jim's brother. Sam and his wife had given up their life in Florida to move in with Jim so that they could take care of him. As I've mentioned, Sam was a bit (well, maybe more than a bit) of a drinker, and I believe he had lived what you might call a pretty sordid past. Despite this, he did a great job of taking care of his father. Given the family conflicts, I reassured Sam often that he was doing a great job and that no matter how hard it got, someday he would look back on this time with gratitude and pride.

So far so good, but there was a catch. Jim's brother lived in the house next door. Sam and his uncle were like oil and water, and clearly had some bad blood between them. There was also tension between Sam and his sister, and Sam and his wife. With all of this conflict simmering, not a meeting went by without some kind of drama. Today was no exception.

Ordinarily, a social worker would handle this kind of meeting, either on her own or in conjunction with me. On this particular occasion no social worker was available, so I was on my own. I don't remember the actual words that were said, but they were many and heated. As sometimes happens, at first the attempt to "communicate" made things worse rather than better. Anger turned to yelling, and yelling to near-blows. Eventually I had to break up what came close to becoming a fist fight. Thanks more to God than to my efforts, no one got hurt. An agreement was finally reached and a truce was called, though neither ended the tension in the family for good.

For years after Jim's death, Sam would call me about once a year or so, always when he had a good alcoholic "buzz" going. It was as though the drinks had freed him up to express things he did not feel comfortable voicing at more lucid times. Sam would speak about how much hospice had done for him and his father, how grateful he was, how right I had been that he would cherish his caregiving when he looked back on it later. These calls were a reminder of what I had realized with sudden clarity on May 2nd: that my work was as much with the families as with the patients themselves. It was also a reminder that no matter what demands or complaints are made in the heat of the moment, neither hospice patients nor families usually expect perfection. None of the many professionals who cared for Jim and his family could permanently "solve" their many issues. In the long run, though, that didn't matter. Sam did not remember the problems, but rather the teamwork, caring and love.

Of course, I had no premonition of this on May 2nd. All I knew that day was that a family boxing match had narrowly been averted. No sooner had I walked from the room in which we had gathered when my pager went off. Yet another interruption: "par for the course" in the day of a hospice nurse.

Roger

The page told me that Roger had just died. I called his girlfriend Cheryl, offered my condolences, and told her I would be there in twenty minutes to make the official pronouncement of death. Over the phone, we both marveled at how accurately he had foretold the day of his passing and shared our gratitude for how peacefully he had died.

I usually keep my eclectic spiritual beliefs quite private. My belief is that we all come from the same God, and that all of the varied ways people acknowledge their divine source should be honored and respected. But I am aware that others may think differently, and always want to honor people wherever they are "at." I also recognize the line between my profession and my personal life.

But on this day, something seemed to demand a different approach. Remembering that I had the sage in my car *and* that I had been guided to put it there, I asked Cheryl if she would like me to smudge Roger (as the burning of the sage is called) at the time of the pronouncement. Commenting that he had recently smudged himself, she said that she would be thrilled. This was a relief to me, and a confirmation that I had truly been spiritually guided.

While driving to do the pronouncement on Roger, I reflected back on the day he told me he was going to die. "I'm going to die on Tuesday," he had told me a few days before. His voice was as matter-of-fact as his words were simple.

"*This* Tuesday?" I felt shock but no disbelief.

"Yup. Two days from today," he said a little smugly.

"How do you know?"

"I dreamed it," he replied.

I had liked Roger from the minute I met him. He was my age, a Vietnam veteran who had a peaceful, calm energy that made him a pleasure to be with. He accepted the coming of his death with grace. I'm not sure whether it was his ten years in Alcoholics Anonymous, his involvement in Native American spiritual traditions, or the combination of the two that helped him reach this emotional place. Whatever it was, he had made peace with his friends, his family, and his life in general, and he felt deeply connected to divine energy and living things.

When I first admitted Roger to hospice, he was living in a single room. The small bathroom attached to it looked like an afterthought. Neither housekeeping nor interior decorating was among his priorities. The only decorations on the dingy grey walls, in fact, were a Native American peace pipe and a poster of Chief Sitting Bull.

Not long after I met him, it became unsafe for Roger to live alone. Reluctantly, he moved into the home of his "significant other," Cheryl. He felt comfortable in his home, however modest it was. Like Roger, many dying patients want to retain their independence and dignity for as long as possible.

The question of how and when to talk about the time and manner of a patient's death can be a tricky one. Many doctors do not feel patients can handle this kind of information, while others blurt it out at times when patients may not be ready for it. Because hospice nurses usually visit more often and interact with patients and families more intimately, we may have a better sense of what is needed. Nine times out of ten, or even ten times out of ten, the patient and family want a sense of the timeframe; there are ways to discuss this potentially complicated information that are helpful, and ways that are less so.

The most important thing we in hospice know is that patients, families, and situations differ greatly. There are many variables in their souls and lives; each person, and each illness, is different. There is no such thing as a certain or accurate answer to most of the questions we are asked. When a patient asks—and only when a patient asks—I will share my "gut" feeling about what their timeframe might be, explaining that it is exactly that. My intuition is based on everything from the indications of the disease, the symptoms and other medical evidence, to my observance of how much the patient is eating, to intangibles like the patient's will and attitude. These latter factors play an enormous role in the end of life, and their importance can't be underestimated.

When I arrived at their home, I made the pronouncement of death for Roger immediately. I then noticed Cheryl's teenaged son was looking a little bewildered and ill at ease. The moments around a death—when there is so much emotion, but not much to do in practical terms—can be difficult, especially for someone young. Knowing that it would be a relief for him to have something to do, I asked him if he had any flute music for our small unofficial ceremony. Looking relieved, he headed for the computer to download something appropriate.

Family and friends had started to gather in the house. Cheryl asked me if I would explain the smudging as I did it. Gathering all ten or so of the people now in the house, we stood in Roger's room. The flute music was playing as I lit the stick of sage. Its sweet-smelling smoke eddied upwards as I explained the significance of the sage and the ceremony.

I smudged Roger and then did each of the others in the room as well. Again to my relief, they all seemed comfortable with the ceremony. It may have been that Roger's friends and family either knew of or shared his commitment to Native American traditions. One of the participants, a co-worker of mine who was also Roger's aunt, was really fascinated by the smudging. The lack of judgment or shock from those in the room was a wonderful blessing. I felt almost as though I had "come out of the closet" with my beliefs, testing my fear of what people might think in the process. But it was the right thing to do for Roger, and this helped me set my concerns aside on this special day.

The ways in which people handle the time after a death varies from family to family and culture to culture. Some families pray, some light a candle, some open a window to allow the spirit to leave. Some family members are comforted to help prepare a body before its passage to a funeral home, while others would be distressed by this task. Often, I can tell without asking what people feel comfortable doing or not doing. But of course, I do ask when necessary, and also listen closely to what friends and family members ask me.

To many people, the task of going to a patient's home and handling the formalities of the pronouncement of death may sound like a sad, depressing, or even frightening part of a hospice nurse's job. For me, it often feels quiet the opposite. I believe it is a great privilege to be there with family and friends at this special moment that is so filled with depth and grace.

Being present with Roger's family after his death was such a moment. So was the pronouncement for my patient Leslie, who suffered from ALS (Lou Gehrig's disease). Leslie was an amazing woman who radiated strength and grace. Even after she lost the ability to speak clearly I continued to feel that we could communicate. I often meditated and prayed for her: asking that she be sent love and light, that she and her family would have clarity about their choices, and that she would go when the time was right. I received the call that she had died only a few hours after one such meditation session. Even the fact that I got that particular call felt like the grace of God: I usually do not have my work cell phone in the house with me when I am not working. Another nurse was on call, but she was tied up many miles away, and thus was delighted to have me do the pronouncement. Leslie's daughter and closest women friends joined me in what turned into a deeply sacred experience. Together, the five of us bathed Leslie's body, shared memories of her and her life through laughter and tears, and agreed that we all felt her spirit—and the holiness of the moment—near us. Leslie's family seemed comforted to learn about my meditation, and that afternoon with them will always remain close to my heart.

Although not everyone agrees, I always feel as though the spirit of the person who has died lingers a while, making the first few hours after a death a blessed time. I usually don't share that belief with a family unless I am specifically asked, but I do handle the actions we all take after a death as though the deceased is aware of them. Hearing has been proven to be the last sense to leave the body, so it makes sense to me that their spirit may be listening or hearing in the time right after death. If Roger's spirit was still in this home, I am glad to know that he was surrounded by love, appreciation for his life, and the beauty of the flute music chosen by Cheryl's son.

Nathan

By now it was close to 5:00 p.m. It was an hour past the official end of my shift, but that was actually less overtime than most days involved. I had one last stop to make before my time with patients and families ended. I don't say "before the workday ended," because there is considerable, time-consuming reporting and paperwork to be done even after all appointments are concluded.

Nathan had been a patient of mine for over a year before being discharged from hospice service. In that time, I had become very close to his wife. I had also worked with two of their daughters years before, so I felt a special connection. As I have said, the boundaries between "patient" and "friend," "nurse" and "friend" can sometimes blur, especially when you work for a long time in the same town or region.

Nathan was a seventy-eight-year-old man with a rare neurological disorder that is often misdiagnosed as Parkinson's disease. In part because of this problem, Nathan was one of those patients who "fell between the cracks" of the medical system. Nathan and his wife Joan had both relied on hospice care. He could no longer speak or control his muscles. It had been hugely comforting to Joan to know that she could rely on twice-daily home health aide visits to help her transfer her husband from bed to chair, and even more reassuring to know that she could pick up the phone and consult a nurse twenty-four hours a day.

However, Nathan's illness became more chronic rather than terminal. As such, it did not allow us to keep him on the hospice service. Each hospice patient must be periodically recertified to establish that he or she still meets hospice criteria. The exact time periods between certifications vary, with Medicare, Medicaid and private insurance each having its own requirements. Nathan simply did not qualify any longer. That should have been good news, at least in theory, as it confirmed that his disease was not terminal at any near date. In Nathan's case, unfortunately, it also meant that Nathan and Joan had to do without the services they depended on to create even a reasonable quality of life—services they could not afford without the financial help provided by hospice certification.

In addition to feeling that the medical system had let Nathan and Joan down, I knew that I would miss my weekly visits to them. Joan absolutely adored this man, to whom she had been married for more than fifty years. She lavished him with love and affection and begrudged not a moment of the twenty-four-hours-a-day care he required. Nathan was himself a smiling, soft-spoken gentleman. His perfectly clean-shaven face and matching beautifully pressed clothing spoke of the pride Joan had in her husband as well as the pride Nathan still felt in himself. Both of them were good, self-reliant people who deserved support on their difficult journey.

Today, Joan and Nathan would probably not have had to cope with the frustrations of being decertified from hospice care. Hospices now offer palliative care programs of a kind that would have been ideal in their situation. I am thrilled that these options exist now, though it saddens me to remember that patients I treated who, like Nathan, were "ahead of their time" where this kind of medical service was concerned.

On an ordinary nursing visit I would have checked Nathan's vital signs, listened to his lung sounds, and worked with Joan to figure out what medications needed to be ordered. After we took care of those practical things, Joan and I would have sat at the kitchen table to share a cup of tea. These times had given her the chance to vent, to share her joys, hopes, worries and pain. I would always encourage her to do what she could to sustain her own strength by getting out of the house or doing something special for herself, but she rarely followed this advice.

On May 2nd, I had no nursing tasks to do. This visit was "off the books," just a personal call to see how Joan and Nathan were managing. I can still remember standing outside Joan's door as I was leaving, encouraging her to write her memoirs. Whether she chose to write about the blessed task of caring for her husband or the painful ways the system let her down, I knew her words would have great power. That is why I shared pieces of my day and felt guided to urge her toward some writing. Now that I am writing *my* book, I can't wait to see if she has written hers.

Top Common Myths about Hospice

1. You have to be actively dying to be signed on to Hospice. The timeframe for signing on to hospice is a physician's expectation that the illness or debility would produce death within six months if it follows its natural course. Many patients live that full six months and many others, as I have noted throughout this book, are actually decertified from hospice care because their life expectancy lengthens beyond the six-month threshold.

2. You have to be homebound to receive hospice care. In fact, if a patient is able, we actually encourage him or her to get out of the home as much as possible, and support families in planning for any travel the patient desires and is able to accomplish. For example, an individual might want to see a certain place or visit with a beloved person before they die. This is all in contrast with VNA service or Palliative Care, which does require that a patient be homebound.

3. A "Do Not Resuscitate" order must be signed in order to receive hospice care. A DNR order allows doctors, nurses, nursing home staff and other medical providers not to intervene, rather than having to take all possible measures to sustain life.

Hospice has no "hard and fast" rule on DNR orders. We welcome our patients and families wherever they are emotionally. Some people are not ready to make the decision to sign a DNR order at the time they sign on to hospice. We respect their feelings and allow them to do whatever they need to make the right decision at the right time.

With that said, we are acutely aware of the benefits of DNR orders and we do encourage them wherever they are appropriate. Lifesaving interventions are usually physically distressing for the patient and emotionally painful for the family. As a hospice nurse, I have seen the toll that is taken on both patient and family when a terminally ill patient in, say, a nursing home setting is repeatedly rushed to a hospital emergency room to be "saved." The additional life span gained is typically short, while the disturbance to quality of life is profound. If a patient is comfortable doing so, signing a DNR allows them to pass on in peace when their time comes, and frees the family of the necessity of watching their loved one subjected to extreme interventions and, perhaps, kept alive in conditions other than those they would wish.

4. Once you are signed onto Hospice you will be drugged with morphine or painkillers. Unlike non-hospice providers, we will prescribe painkillers as required to make a patient comfortable, without refusing them on grounds such as fear of future addiction, and morphine is among the medications that may be used. However, pain medication is neither a universal norm nor a necessity. We want patients to have the best possible quality of life—and that means as little medication of any kind, and as much ordinary alertness and awareness, as is feasible. Morphine will only be suggested if the patient requires it for serious pain or shortness of breath. Even then, and as is true with all drugs, our motto is always "start low and go slow."

5. Once someone is on morphine under Hospice care, the end is near. It is true that morphine lowers the respiratory threshold, causing a person to take fewer, deeper breaths than they would otherwise. However, acknowledging this is not the same as saying that morphine use equals death! Like virtually every other drug and treatment, morphine produces different results in different situations. Many people who are prescribed it go to work and live a normal life thanks to its powerful pain-relieving properties. When it comes to hospice patients, it's all the more beneficial to let go of any sense of stigma about using it. I always tell patients to "make friends with morphine" when the situation warrants.

6. Once signed up for hospice, a patient's ordinary, existing medications are stopped. This is not so. Medications and treatments that support a patient's comfort and quality of life are continued, and may even be enhanced.

7. You need to have cancer to be signed on to Hospice. Any illness or condition that, given its natural course may result in death within six months or less, qualities a patient for Hospice. Cancer is among the most common of these, but far from the only one.

8. Patients in nursing homes or other specialized facilities are not eligible for hospice care. As noted elsewhere in this book, this is not true. A patient can be in a nursing home or even some hospitals and still be treated under hospice protocols.

9. Hospice will provide 24-hour-a-day care. The distinction here is subtle but crucial. Hospice is *on call* 24 hours a day, but does not *provide care* 24 hours a day. (The only exceptions occur in hospices that offer either in-hospital hospice care or their own hospice houses—but these situations *are* exceptions.) Our role is to provide the specialized services family and friends do not have the training to offer, while teaching those same family and friends to provide more routine kinds of care a dying person needs.

10. Hospice means a pain-free death. The most comfortable and painless death possible is always our goal, and hospices are armed with a wide variety of strategies to minimize pain and maximize comfort. Yet there are some things no provider can control. Every so often, no matter what we do, a patient may die in pain. This is surely the exception rather than the rule, but it does happen.

For me, the best consolation is to know that in the great majority of cases, a person's death is at least *more* comfortable under Hospice than without our involvement. Whether it is the right mix of medication...an aide who keeps the patient clean and comfortable...a nurse who helps answer the family's questions about the dying process...a chaplain to offer spiritual care...a volunteer who gives family caregivers respite...or the support of a social worker in the midst of complex family conflicts, Hospice help does much to make dying as easy for both patient and family as possible, even when some pain is involved.

Part Two: The Journey of a Hospice Nurse

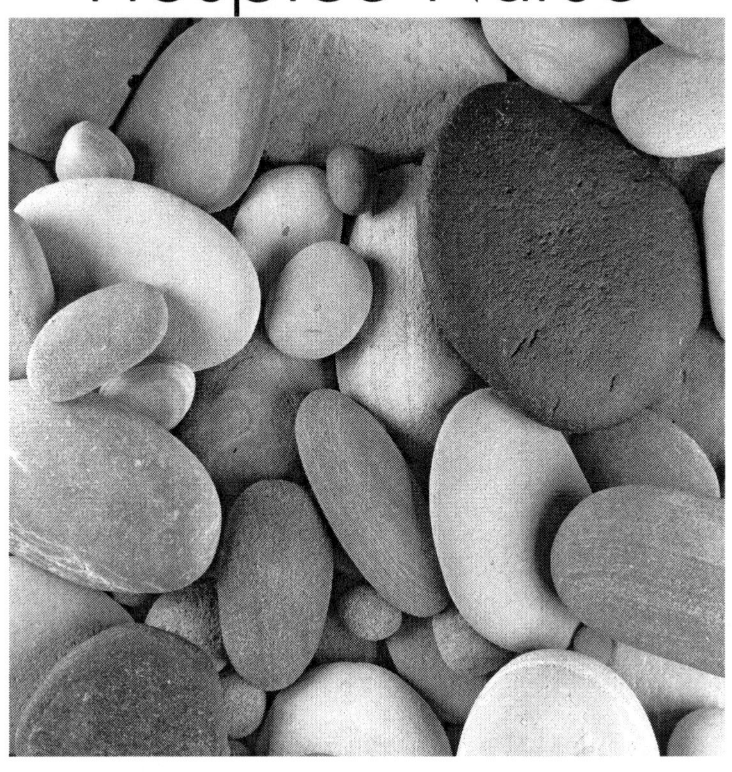

All healing is essentially the release from fear.
—A Course in Miracles

A Journey Begins

Those of us who work with, for, or around hospice—either professionally or as volunteers—are a diverse lot. The journeys that bring us to hospice are varied, colorful, sometimes dramatic, sometimes painful. What most of us share is some kind of strong sense that we are called to this particular work. That calling can come in the form of personal experience with loss or death...a spiritual mission...a path of professional growth or challenge. Whatever it looks like, it is the answer to the question we are so frequently asked, "How can you do such sad, difficult work?" For me and many of my colleagues, the explanation is "simply" that we know it is *our* work, our mission. And, for that reason, it does not—at least usually—feel unbearably hard or difficult to us, but rather fulfilling and inspirational.

The next few chapters of this book tell the story of my journey as seen through three different perspectives: that of my conventional education, my spiritual growth, and my learning about holistic healing. I want to emphasize, before I begin, that I am not telling my story because I believe that I am in any way exceptional or important. Instead, I tell it as a way of illustrating how many different paths—and how many different stops on those paths—can lead to hospice work. Those of us who work in hospice are just as human as anyone else; just as prone to stumbles and surprises, hard decisions and unexpected detours; and just as grateful for the grace which shows us the way forward.

Nothing in my childhood suggested that I would gravitate toward, much less enjoy, higher education. As I have mentioned before, I grew up in a very small town in Maine. It was called New Vineyard, and at the time it had a population of approximately five hundred residents. Of course, a town this small had an equally small school. The first school I ever attended was a two-room schoolhouse. Classes for all of the grades from first through fourth were held in one room, classes for fifth through eighth grades in the room across the hall. I guess you could say that this schooling qualifies me as "a hick from the sticks."

When I was in the second grade, my family moved to the next town over. Farmington had a population of about seven thousand. To someone like me, this new home seemed like a bustling metropolitan city.

I adjusted fairly well to the change, as far as I can recall. But the next year, my mother gave birth to my baby sister, Christine. Christine lived for only two days. During my mother's pregnancy, I had prayed that she would die, because I didn't want to give up my position as the baby of the family. From my point of view, I already had a sister who was three years older than I was, and that was quite sufficient in terms of family size. Naturally, when Christine died I felt I had caused her death—and I felt overwhelming guilt as a result. My training has since taught me that children often feel responsible for bad things that occur to, or in, their families. Feelings of responsibility, guilt, and shame are even more common when it comes to the death of siblings, for whom a child will normally have ambivalent feelings of love and resentment. Of course, I had no way of knowing how normal I was back then.

I'm not sure exactly how long I carried this guilt around in silence. Fortunately, I finally found the courage to speak. I can still picture myself sitting in my mother's lap at the kitchen table, explaining to her that Christine's death was my fault. I was young enough that I now can't recall her words exactly, but I remember her love and warmth clearly. Without a moment's judgment or hesitation she explained that Christine had died as a result of medical complications and that I had absolutely nothing to do with her death. Her words seemed to lift the weight of the world off my shoulders. I thank God that I was able to express my fears to my mother and that she was able to hear me so completely, even though she must have been struggling with her own grief as well.

Though it had felt large to me as a child, Farmington was not a stimulating place for a maturing teenager. We had a single movie theater, for example, which (unlike today's multi-plexes) showed just one film each week. School dances, though they were few and far between, were a major social event. Without any chance to travel or explore the world, without even the computers that make today's teenagers feel connected to life outside their community, I often felt restless and bored.

My best friend during those years was Vicki DePue, who had moved to Farmington from California in the third grade. We were inseparable "partners in crime," and also the first and pretty much the only hippies in town. We got the first wire-framed glasses to appear in our school, and were the only two students to go to Woodstock. Beyond that, our idea of a good time was to get a six-pack of beer and sneak into a school alcove that perfectly echoed the obnoxious sounds we made.

Vicki helped lessen the persistent feeling that I was a misfit or oddball that dogged my entire adolescence in Farmington. The feeling of being "out of step" with the world is especially painful for teenagers, because they don't yet know how many other—and very different—possible places and lifestyles await them. Vicki helped me survive that pain, which lasted for many years. Without her, I'm not sure I could have survived adolescence in Farmington. She was the kind of friend that only comes around once in a lifetime. Sadly, Vicki died at the age of only twenty-five. She had brittle diabetes, which interacted with a heroin overdose. Vicki used to come to me in dreams quite often, but I have not "seen" her in years now.

During my high school years, an aunt who lived not far from us had a leg amputated in her early forties. Over my school vacation I spent every day at her bedside. Her four children made brief visits, but I was the only one who felt comfortable doing the kind of nursing care she needed. Managing things like bathing, rubdowns, and the bedpan seemed natural to me—a part of life and love, not an onerous duty. I had never consciously wanted to be a nurse—in fact, when my peers spoke of their dreams of teaching or nursing, I remember wanting to run an orphanage! Still, I think it was at this time that the nursing seed was planted in my heart.

My grades in high school were shameful at best. School didn't come easy to me. Today, I understand that I learn best in experience-based programs and perform best in classes that rely more on written work and essay exams than on traditional "cut and dried" formats such as multiple choice testing. Back then, such differences in learning style were never discussed—at least, never discussed with me! Upon graduating from high school, I swore that I would never be caught dead in a school again.

Despite all this, in 1971, I found myself enrolled in a nursing diploma program. I chose to return to a school that was hands-on in its teaching. It was also affordable enough for me to pay for myself rather than asking my parents for the money. The program at the Worcester City Hospital School of Nursing was based on learning by experience, which would ordinarily be my strong suit. However, I have to admit that my personal life, which you could say was colorful, was a considerable distraction. My boyfriend at the time robbed a bank during the three years I was in the program. With the proceeds he bought me a yellow Triumph convertible, explaining that he couldn't stand to see me hitchhike to and from school. I spent the next year visiting him in a variety of prisons. Not surprisingly, this episode nearly got me expelled from the school.

These bumps in the road notwithstanding, I graduated from the program in 1974. Wanting to experience life in a different and more exciting place, I applied for and got my first nursing job in California. The position at Sequoia Hospital in Redwood City came with an in-depth orientation to the Intensive Care unit, Cardiac Care unit, and Transitional Care unit. I learned a tremendous amount about tending to the critically or terminally ill during this time.

I also got my first introduction to meditation while I worked at the hospital. (I talk about this experience in more detail in a later chapter.) Beginning to meditate on a regular basis opened up a whole new world for me. Soon, meditation alone wasn't enough. I began to explore holistic healing modalities, soaking them up like a human sponge. From Transcendental Meditation, I went on to study Swedish Eselan massage, tai chi, and Touch for Health, to name just a few. I was attracted to the healing power of crystals and did some laying on of stones.

The people I met during this journey of learning were a kind of revelation to me. For the first time in my life I was around like-minded people, people who did not see me or my curiosity as being weird, people who like me were seekers and explorers. What a gift it is to discover that you *do* fit in!

Toni, my best friend in California, was also a huge influence in my life at this time. She was a native Californian who seemed to know all the local facts and lore that I did not. So she was able to orient this country bumpkin from conservative New England into the ways of this new, hip state. I remember her telling me on the day we met that "San Francisco is called 'the city,' not 'Frisco'. Women are women, not 'chicks.' And African Americans are 'blacks,' not 'Negroes.'" These 'tips' sound rather trivial, but like her friendship, they helped me feel at home in my new world. In the end, I spent six years as a resident of the Bay Area. These years were rich with learning, growing, evolving and exploring for me.

Toni and I later quit excellent jobs to volunteer after an earthquake destroyed much in Guatemala. Our poor Spanish got us "bumped" from the program, but since we no longer had work, we decided we might as well do some travel anyway. We made a three-week trip through Mexico, a journey that was more radical than it may seem today (it was not considered to be safe at the time and our Spanish left much to be desired). Our limited funds made third-class travel a must. If you truly want to see the reality of a place, this is the way to go, as it immediately brings you "up close and personal" with everything from the landscape, the villages, the people, and even the livestock!

A year later, Toni and I both signed up for tutoring classes in Guatemala. The classes were slated to last for a month, but before coming home, I ran off to Tikal, one of the Seven Wonders of the World, with a man I had met. The experiences of that trip were like scenes out of the movie "Deliverance" with a little bit of "The African Queen" mixed in: slinging a hammock up in the jungle, hitching rides through the banana groves, hiring a boat to rescue us after we were stranded along the river, where all roads ended and only jungle remained. The man I was with spoke fluent Spanish, which allowed me to immerse myself in the experience. My own Spanish leaves much to be desired to this day, but in every other way the experience was the trip of a lifetime.

The second step program I attended at Sonoma State University in Rohnert Park, California was another life changing experience. Because I was a California resident, my tuition was paid for and books were the main cost of my education. At that time, the University had a flexible program. I was able to write my own curriculum as to what I would take and how I would get graded. Now that I was free of the financial burden that college usually imposes *and* free to choose classes, like those in holistic health, which truly interested me, I loved school. The days when I "wouldn't be caught dead going back to school" were long—and permanently—gone.

I heard the word "Hospice" first during this time. The memory of my experience in the lake as a child came back to me, and I immediately knew I was destined to be part of this growing movement. Choosing to do my preceptorship with hospice; I had the opportunity to take workshops with extraordinary experts like Elizabeth Kübler-Ross and Stephen Levine. What a gift it was to sit and learn with people like this.

In the end, my time at Sonoma State affected me personally as well as professionally. In my "Death and Dying" class, we were asked to imagine that we had only six months to live and then write about how we would spend that time. This exercise forced me to focus intensely on my priorities—to picture a situation in which there was no chance to explore all of the many things in life that interested and attracted me. To my surprise, what I wanted to do with this precious time was spend it with Richard, a man I had met back East, during a visit home. Feeling so drawn to a person I had only known a month rather than, say, my family or old friends startled me. Suddenly I was aware of how much I loved this man. I asked him to marry me, and he said "yes." We've been together ever since. Given what I have shared about previous boyfriends, I should add that Richard was a *much* better selection!

Richard had a construction business in Massachusetts. As much as I loved California, it didn't make sense for him to move his work there. I was clearly the one who had more flexibility. In deciding to move back to New England, I felt that I could use some time to digest the huge amount of information I had "inhaled" in California before picking up my work or education again.

I did need a breather, a time to pause and reflect. But what I hadn't factored in was how life takes over the best-laid plans. Rather than returning promptly to my search for truth and vocation, I had first one, then another, daughter. With a family to care for and all the other demands of "real life," it was much more complicated to change course, like I had when I was young and single. In the end, it would take more than twelve years and some tough life lessons before I returned to the work of finding and embracing my authentic self.

New Directions

For many years, I thought that I lost my identity while my daughters were growing up. Being a mother is certainly all-consuming, but when I reflect back today I see that this belief isn't accurate. My passions and interests never disappeared entirely. One example of this, which still makes me proud, is my commitment to educating my daughters—and their friends and classmates—in healthy and eco-friendly living.

Each year from first grade through sixth grade, I spent Earth Day in their classrooms talking about ways to honor the Earth and become more environmentally conscious. This all sounds pretty "ho hum" today, but at the time it was quite unusual. The term "green" and the fashion for environmental activism did not yet exist. Those of us who saw Earth as a living being or advocated for natural-foods diets definitely stuck out…in fact, my children's classmates still remember me as "the Earth Day lady." The impact of these efforts might have been minimal. I know that my own kids, for example, always tried to trade their healthy lunches for the junk food they could not get at home! But the intention and belief were there, proving that while my values had gotten somewhat submerged during these years, they never disappeared.

As the girls got older, though, my sense that I was not living a fully authentic life grew stronger. I have since spoken to many other women who share this same experience. Having changed their course to focus on their families, they may feel lost as their children become more independent. It feels "selfish" to turn the focus back to ourselves, and scary to try to jump-start careers that have been on hold for years, maybe decades.

For me, as for many of these other women, the result is depression. My bouts with clinical depression taught me how different clinical depression is from merely feeling sad or blue. The feeling is overwhelming, exhausting, isolating, and intractable. I tried talk therapy, which did not work. Nor was medication the answer. Frustrated and confused, I really doubted my sanity at times. Eventually, I decided to become my own healer instead.

I began by learning Neuro-Linguistic Programming, or NLP. This modality was considered very "cutting edge" at the time. Working with Dr. Richard Clark, one of the founding fathers of the technique, was a profound pleasure and privilege. A Zen master for over thirty years and a former neurochemist, Dr. Clark was gentle and wise. As always, being around mentors like this and immersing myself in learning was both healing and life-altering.

After some time in this program, I found myself torn. One option was to pursue my training with NLP and go for certification as a hypnotherapist. The other was to enter graduate school for a program in counseling. I eventually chose the latter, motivated partly by my long-held desire to move out of nursing as a career. The lack of collegiality in nursing had disturbed me from the beginning. There seemed to be an atmosphere of competition and back-stabbing rather than a commitment to mutual support and growth. I would eventually learn that hospice nurses are an exception in this regard. They feel like family, and my dialogue with fellow hospice nurses has never been anything but mutually supportive and encouraging. However, I hadn't yet learned about this, so I entered a satellite graduate program offered by Leslie College out of Cambridge, Massachusetts.

The program ran for two and a half years. It met one weekend per month at a location in Hatfield, Mass. The flexible, low-residency structure met my needs perfectly. I could work part-time, attend school, and be there for my family—an ideal situation. The groups were small and, as a result, close; the instructors were innovative and open. By allowing me to write papers that built on my personal experiences rather than abstract factual information, the teachers allowed me to learn in a way that was comfortable for me, as well as to explore the emotional challenges I had recently faced. In the course of these studies, my depression lifted. In that sense, returning to the learning I loved allowed me to be my own therapist.

Just prior to entering Leslie College, I had discovered a holistic nursing program called Seeds and Bridges. Now known as the Birchtree Healing Center, this program offered exactly the kind of rich, spirit-nurturing mental and emotional "food" I had been needing for so long. The first session I attended was in Salem, Massachusetts. I sat in a circle surrounded by forty nurses from all over the country. The knowledge that I was among like-minded souls gave me the feeling of coming home. It was one of the most affirming and supportive experiences of my entire nursing career. In fact, it was this program that helped rekindle the passion for nursing I thought I had lost forever.

To my delight, I was able to incorporate this holistic nursing program with my graduate work. Spirituality was the common thread that ran through both. Focusing on this theme felt authentic and inspiring to me. I developed a spirituality group in a locked psychiatric unit and wrote a research proposal on spirituality and psychotherapy. My final thesis was entitled "Depression and The Power of Prayer." I graduated in 1997 with the feeling that I was finally back on track. My first subsequent job was as a psych nurse with a small VNA/Hospice. I became the Bereavement Coordinator, then the Volunteer Coordinator. Eventually, I found my way to hospice nursing, which I have practiced ever since.

I would never have been able to do this demanding and unpredictable form of nursing when my children were small. It is too all-consuming and unpredictable. With the girls growing up, however, it fit perfectly. Hospice nursing brings together so many of my passions: my sense of death as a profound and holy transition, my love for healing and helping, and my reverence for the power of spirituality of all kinds. Very soon after I began my service as a hospice nurse I knew I had found my life's work, my true calling. The sense of unrest I had always felt was gone; I had truly come home.

When I am sitting with a patient and their family, explaining hospice and signing them on to our service, I feel completely at peace. There is nowhere else I would rather be and nothing else that I would rather be doing. I feel a love, compassion, commitment and reverence that nurture me as well as my patients.

Connecting with people at this deep soul level and helping them make the transition from this life to the next is special work—God's work. Facing death is a humbling experience, a powerful reminder of how precious life is and how little the everyday distractions, regrets, and "drama" really means. Dealing with death every day makes it so much easier to focus on the miracles and synchronicities—*Godincidences*, as Maya Angelou would say—that surround us. I believe that you cannot do this work without learning how to live life more fully and be grateful for what you have. I feel so blessed to take part in it. My work with hospice helps me see God in each and every being, and to live my life richly, as if each day were my last.

Spiritual Paths

Like my education in nursing, hospice, and holistic healing, my spiritual journey has been a long and eclectic one, which has taken me down many roads. What church (if any) I was attending and how I was feeling about it varied hugely over the years. But two things have never really changed at all. The first is my sense that spirituality is not some narrow religious denomination or set of specific rules, but rather a deep connection both to a divine source and to all other life forms. I once came across a journal article that defined spirituality in a way that really resonated. Its authors, Jacobson and Burnhart, called spirituality "a sense of harmonious interconnectedness between self, others, nature and the Ultimate Other, which exists throughout and beyond time and space."

- The second consistent thread in my spirituality is my sense of the sacred connection between all aspects of my life's purpose. For me, there is no separation between my work in hospice, my work in holistic modalities, and my spirituality. All of these melt together in a single holy "pot." Whatever affects one aspect affects the others as well.

My first experiences with religion were not very comfortable ones. My parents never attended church themselves, but they insisted that my sister and I go to the Baptist church every Sunday. I even sang in the choir—not exactly a heavenly experience, as my tone-deafness forced the choir director to ask me to lip-synch. I liked the robes and the chance to be in the "spotlight," but the services confused me. I didn't understand them, and I absolutely hated the "yelling."

When I was a teenager, the Episcopal Church got a new, hip priest. My sister and I found that church much more appealing, for obvious though not very spiritual reasons. But I found myself having unaccountable fits of inappropriate laughter. I was glad when I graduated from high school and the need for church attendance ceased. After that, I stayed out of churches for many years. I just didn't see what they could offer me, and I had no beliefs that seemed to fit with their creeds.

It wasn't until my late twenties that my interest in religion surfaced. As is not unusual in my life, it happened in a way that was unexpected at best. My girlfriend Mary and I were driving from California to Maine in a pick-up truck. Two women in hiking boots with waist-length hair and California license plates were naturally a "red flag" near the Buffalo, New York border. When we were asked if we were carrying drugs, Mary blurted out that she had some peyote. She had actually been carrying it for years, waiting for the right moment to use it; we had thought that if we happened to visit a Native American reservation, it might be a spiritual experience. As it turned out, the right time for that peyote would never come. Possessing this hallucinogen was a Class A felony, and we were promptly arrested. *TWO NURSES BAGGED AT BORDER*, the local headlines screamed.

What followed was like something out of a fictional novel or adventurous movie. We spent one long night in jail before being taken under the wing of a female police officer who was planning to become a nun. She managed to get us released to the care of the Convent of the Sisters of Mercy in Buffalo, New York. Our first night there, the sisters took us to the chapel, where they played the guitar and sang songs like "It's a Long Road to Freedom" and "Working on a Chain Gang." During our stay there we took calls from lawyers about our case, got asked by other convents to speak to their postulants, took Mass with the priest and circle of nuns using French bread and wine, and, I must admit, taught the nuns and several priests to do tequila shots with lemon and salt. Only in the 1970s, I guess.

I was surprised by many of the nuns. Here, to my surprise—in a place where I would have expected narrow minds or judgment—I found spiritual depth, openness and curiosity. One of the sisters, who was working on a doctorate in theology, explained to me that meditation was listening to God, while prayer was talking to God. Finally, some part of organized religion made sense to me. For what was really the first time, I could understand why a church or religious practice would be worth seeking out.

After this experience, I actively sought a church to attend. Unfortunately, my first adult experiences with churches were as disappointing as my childhood ones had been. The Christian churches I tried saw my reverence for the Earth and all life forms, which I had learned from the Native American tradition, as being somehow pagan. Having a crucial part of my spirituality deemed inconsistent with Christianity created a major struggle for me. It took many years to find a church that resonated with my beliefs and welcomed me just as I was.

The first church that ever truly fed my spiritual hunger was the Glide Memorial Chapel in San Francisco. Whether this was due to its location, its congregation, or its pastor, the Chapel was a place of openness, affirmation and joy. Its pastor, Cecil Williams, was a dynamic black man who had been the mediator during the Patti Hurst hostage negotiations in the 1960s. Not surprisingly, he was fearless, inspiring, full of energy, and uninterested in petty rules. The services always featured songs from the artists of the day and participants from all over the world. I never walked out of that church without feeling lifted and filled by the Holy Spirit. Even my parents, who were so much more traditional than I was, were moved when they went to a service with me during their first visit to California. We left hugging and crying, filled with love.

There were no churches like Glide Memorial available nearby when my daughters were young. Richard and I wanted them to have a foundation of faith, so I began attending St. Philip's Episcopal Church in Easthampton, Mass. Richard's grandparents were married there in 1926, so I had a feeling of having some roots there. For twenty years

I acted as a lay Eucharistic minister, administering communion. This ritual spoke to me more than anything else in the faith.

A recent experience gave me the sense that I had somehow come full circle from my early days in California. I was at the Omega Institute in Rhinebeck, New York, taking a workshop on energy medicine. Donna Eden, the practitioner, bases her work on Touch for Health, which she learned in Northern California in the mid-1970s, exactly as I did. For all I know, we may have been in some of the same classes. I was never very good at the muscle testing that is the basis for this system. It is too delicate, and too easy a target for critics and nay-sayers. My father was a skeptic who tended to ridicule things, making me sensitive to this. My husband is a skeptic as well, so I guess I have tended to stay "in the closet" on such matters all these years.

For this reason, I have welcomed the greater openness to mind/body/spirit connections that has finally come to the Northeast, where I live. It is wonderful to see more and more like-minded people working in and around the health care and hospice systems. In terms of my own spiritual journey, I continue to meditate—daily when possible, as often as I can when things get hectic. I am currently exploring new churches in my area. I am also hosting a Course in Miracles group, which is filled with amazing women. Our regular meetings are times of joy, deep learning, and reflection.

My work in hospice continues to feed my spirituality. As I have commented before, doing hospice work is the closest you can get to spirit while here on the Earth plane. My experience has been that as people prepare to make the transition from this life into the next, a change takes place. It is as if the soul is preparing to leave the physical body and return to the spiritual realm. Those of us who work with people at these times are familiar with the changes. We always know when someone is getting close to death. Many of the dying report seeing family or friends who have preceded them from this life to the next. The closer you come to the spirit world, the closer the spirit world comes to you. When I ask a patient if they have seen or heard from any deceased family and friends and they say yes, I know their time is getting closer. Skeptics believe it is the narcotics speaking, or perhaps just a dream, but we in hospice know how real it is.

I recently attended a weekend at Omega facilitated by John Holland, Brian Weiss, Raymond Moody and Suzanne Northrup. Entitled *Soul Survival*, the workshop confirmed my belief about connections between the spirit and earthly worlds. John Holland, a medium of amazing skill and integrity, explained his work in a way that enlightened and fascinated me. He described how he increases his vibration, or frequency, through meditation and other means, while the spirits on the other side lower their vibration or frequency so that the two can meet in the middle. Physicians or scientists reading this may be shaking their heads, but it makes perfect sense to me. It seems to be the same process my patients are experiencing when they are preparing to pass on. Raising our vibration is also the same basic principle many of us use when meditating. I personally use a Tibetan bowl or Egyptian healing rods to lift my vibration when I am working to manifest something in my life or trying to enhance my meditation or prayer.

John Holland also taught that those who have passed on communicate with loved ones through pennies and electrical pathways such as radio or TV. He joked that they must be cheap, as they clearly prefer pennies to larger coins; the husband of my dear friend and former supervisor seems to be an exception, as he has "sent" her dimes since the day he died. Most of us who work in hospice have heard thousands of accounts of ways in which deceased loved ones have communicated: through visions, electricity, smells, touch, nature…the list goes on and on.

Because our society is so uncomfortable with death and dying, most people are reluctant to speak about either. As a result, we don't always help each other deal with, talk about, or face loss. Given that death is inevitable, I'm always amazed by this "mental block" in our otherwise very open culture, and grateful that hospice creates a place where conversations on these matters can be shared. The chaplain for our hospice, Carole Schulte, had powerful words to say on this one day recently as we sat together.

We all walk this life for a reason. We all have our own pathway. As a hospice team, our mission is to walk that pathway with [our patients]: to honor and respect their path, and help them live their time in the way they need to live, and not impose what we think they need. In understanding hospice, we can offer people a lens to look at life differently. For example, we can help them ask, how do I want to live my life? What do I still want to do? Who do I need to make amends with? Who do I need to forgive? How do I want to be remembered? What is the legacy that I want to leave? In hospice, we have the opportunity to open doors for people. Hospice is symbolic of what life can be.

She and I agree that hospice is in our blood…a crucial piece of who we are. This sentiment is almost certainly shared by many if not most of those who also do this work. As we sipped our tea, Carol went on to say how differently we would view our lives if we knew how profound and precious both we and life itself are. As Carol says,

I believe that Cicely Saunders, the founder of hospice, was divinely inspired during her search to alleviate suffering. Spiritual pain encompasses all pain; soul searching, making peace with your life, and letting go of it… there is a whole level of discernment that must be learned and practiced.

Spirituality is for everyone; religion may or may not be. Those who have a religion do not necessarily adhere to it, while those who belong to no "official" faith may feel deeply connected to the divine. Feelings of guilt and judgment affect everyone. Many people grow up with a vision of a vengeful, punishing God. In hospice we try to help patients heal those broken places.

Everyone is afraid to die to some extent, whether their fear is the fear of the unknown, fear of being alone, or fear of pain. Our job in hospice is to offer a compassionate presence as we enter this sacred space with the patient and his or her family. Being at peace with the end of life does not depend on belief or religion per se. It happens when people feel good about their lives. If they have had love, they have peace in their hearts. People who feel connected to something greater than themselves—whether it be God, the universal life force, love—often find death easier, perhaps because they trust more deeply in the natural and spiritual cycle.

Exploring Holistic Healing

As I have mentioned throughout this book, I have been interested in complementary healing modalities throughout my career. I should say right here that while many people refer to this category of medicine as "alternative" healing, I typically avoid that term, as I do not like the "either/or" choice it implies. The term "complementary," which suggests an array of possibilities, is far more accurate. Though it has taken a long time for the profession to accept, much less embrace, non-Western approaches, patients today have a far wider range of options than was the case when my first training occurred. In ideal situations they can benefit from the "best of both worlds," using the Western *and* non-traditional techniques that benefit them, together in a complementary fashion.

Before I discuss some of the holistic modalities and my experience with them, I want to clarify two issues. First, the patient's permission is "job one." It is never my practice to work complementary techniques on a patient who is uncomfortable with them in any way. I may do a bit of silent prayer on my own, but beyond that I always ask a patient if they are interested in trying something new before I begin.

Consistent with that, intention is key when working with complementary healing modalities. Much of Western medicine can be practiced simply by turning on a machine, running a test, or prescribing a pill. Little focus or attention on the practitioner's part is required. Most complementary systems are completely different. They require a practitioner who is clear, fully present, and centered in a healing intention.

This is one of the reasons I often pray silently while caring for patients. In addition to its other benefits, the prayer keeps my intention focused and my energy field clear. It is very easy to take in a patient's energetic, emotional or other disturbance if you are not conscious of the potential for energy "overlap." Conversely, I truly believe that something almost magical happens when energy is exchanged with the intention for deep healing. Healing can take on many forms, not all of which involve a "cure." One of the things I love about complementary modalities is the way they benefit both the recipient and the practitioner him- or herself.

The first, pivotal experience in my education in holistic modalities occurred during my first nursing job in Redwood City, California. A patient who had been horribly injured in an automobile accident came through our Emergency Room. This woman had suffered multiple rib fractures, a broken arm, and a punctured lung. She arrived at the ER with less than a pint of blood circulating through her system. The doctors who saw her were in awe that she was not only still alive, but also conscious, coherent and calm.

The explanation for this remarkable resilience turned out to be that she was experienced in meditation. Knowing that she was alone and seriously injured when the accident happened, she went into a meditative state while waiting and praying for help to arrive. What an extraordinary demonstration of meditation's capacity to affect not just our minds but our bodies. I'm pretty sure that every doctor, nurse, orderly and janitor in the ER and critical care units, if not in the entire hospital, signed up for Transcendental Meditation classes that week!

Her recuperation in the hospital continued to prove meditation's powers. When her friends visited, they would form a circle around her, hold hands, and go into meditation. As caregivers on the floor watched her monitoring equipment with fascination, her blood pressure, pulse and respiration would drop and steady with what seemed like miraculous speed.

Naturally, this fascinated me and my co-workers. We began to spend breaks trying out this new tool. We would take turns meditating while hooked up to various monitors. It took some of us a while, but we could eventually learn to control our bodies' responses with our minds.

Meeting this extraordinary woman was a pivotal point in my life, as well as in the lives of many of the others who had the privilege of knowing her. She was an accomplished musician, who had once performed with Andy Williams. More importantly, she was what I can only call an enlightened being, with a wonderful aura of grace around her. I could see that meditation, among other tools, had focused, quieted and strengthened her soul as well as helping to save and heal her body. It had changed her life, and I knew I wanted it to change mine as well. As I've mentioned earlier, I still meditate regularly, a practice that makes a tremendous difference to my life.

In terms of patient work, my primary holistic practice these days is reflexology. Anyone who has ever had a full body massage probably remembers the wonderful feeling of having their feet massaged. Reflexology can feel something like that, although it involves much more than massage. Instead, it is based on the Chinese system of the energy meridians that run through the body. The meridians end in the feet, where there are reflex points which correspond to all of the major organs and systems. As is true with a number of holistic approaches, reflexology is not typically considered a diagnostic tool or, usually, a "cure." Rather, it is a way to promote balance. It can reduce stress, promote relaxation, improve circulation, release toxins, and revitalize energy. I'm sure I don't have to explain how helpful all of these benefits can be to someone who is seriously ill or dying.

I first began to study this technique in California. Though I was a nurse at the time, I worked for a short time through an agency which needed health aides more than nurses. As an aide in a hospital, I had the time to learn and practice the art of reflexology. Two women who shared a room were receptive to my help in this regard. One was in her seventies, the other only nineteen. Both were very constipated. This certainly isn't a glamorous symptom, and it usually doesn't sound very serious to those of us who are healthy. In actuality, it is a common and very uncomfortable problem for those who are ill, bedridden, and/or on narcotics. Laxatives sometimes work to help relieve the condition, but are often invasive, uncomfortable, unpredictable, and embarrassing.

I stood by these women's beds and worked the heels and arches of their feet, the areas associated with the colon. Lo and behold, when I returned the following night both reported that the treatment had worked. I was given the credit and called "the foot lady" by many of the hospital staff. While other factors may have played a part, reflexology continues to offer help with this same symptom in my hospice work today.

One patient I remember vividly had a hugely distended belly, referred to as ascities, which is the buildup of fluid in the abdomen caused by her liver cancer. Soap-sud enemas had been the only way she was able to move her bowels prior to my visits, and they were very painful for her. I asked her if she would be open to having me try reflexology on her—a question I always ask before even thinking of doing this kind of work. She said yes, and we gave it a try. She never needed an enema after that point. She would marvel at the benefit and joke that she was going to take a picture of her "results." The thought of me going on vacation or being out sick even worried her. Clearly, she was my "success story."

After thirty years of using reflexology only to alleviate constipation, I decided to broaden my learning with further certification. I trained in 2005 at the Omega Institute, which I have mentioned previously. The program required work hours as well as class time. Two of my hospice patients, both women who were in a local nursing home, volunteered to participate, giving me the "hands on" practice I needed to complete the course.

Ella was a woman in her seventies, who I believe had pancreatic cancer. During our first session, she remarked on tenderness when I pressed on the point of her foot that is correlated to the sciatic nerve. When I asked if she had sciatica, she was startled. "How did you know that? Just today, my sciatica starting acting up, but I haven't told a soul!" I am not sure that Ella believed in reflexology before this, but she certainly did from then on. Her sciatic pain did not return, though this was the exception in terms of reflexology's benefits rather than the rule. As noted above, it is not generally considered a "cure." In addition to sciatica, Ella had chronic lower back pain and chronic constipation. She reported relief from both as a result of our sessions.

Laura was in her forties, with tumors that had metastasized to the bone. Being bedridden, she also had pressure sores on her coccyx. Both of these gave her substantial pain, but her desire to be awake and alert for her family made her reluctant to take the full allowable dosage of the narcotics that could alleviate her discomfort.

Laura's husband and daughter were utterly devoted to her. They were by her side at all times except when I made my visits. At those times, she would dismiss everyone, nursing staff included, from her private room. She even made a sign for her door warning people not to disturb her during our appointments and the half hour or so afterward. I felt so grateful to be able to give her some relief. We both enjoyed the visits, which were relaxing enough for her that she would often drift off to sleep before I tiptoed away. I remember her courage, her dedication to her family and her beautiful feet! Her daughter attended to them, keeping her mom perfectly pedicured with freshly painted toenails.

Family members often feel terribly helpless in the face of a loved one's terminal illness. They are thrilled to have something to do to help. I gave Laura's daughter a simplified lesson about the reflex points so that Laura could benefit from some reflexology when I was not there and her daughter could feel there was something to do that would help her mom.

Watching holistic practices or practitioners at work can be very helpful to hospital or facility staff. Even those who may not feel open to complementary modalities sometimes become interested when they see beneficial results being produced. The nurses at Laura and Ella's nursing home requested an "in service" session from me (I am ashamed to say that I never got around to doing it). This lapse notwithstanding, I love to share these techniques with others just as much as I love to learn new modalities myself. There is little time for much in the way of holistic work in the course of a hospice nursing visit. There is so much else to attend to, and so little time. I try to do what reflexology I can, which tends to make my home visits longer than those of some of the other nurses. One of my professional goals is to work even more extensively with holistic modalities, especially by providing training that could help others incorporate those practices into their end-of-life care.

In addition to reflexology, I am a reiki practitioner. Reiki is perhaps the most subtle of the complementary modalities. While it is typically practiced by putting one's hands gently on the recipient, it does not actually require touch or even physical presence. It can be done anywhere, at any time. It works through the joining of the life force between the universe, the practitioner and the recipient. This sounds impossible to many people, but—along with many others—I have seen its tangible results. It is very relaxing, and many recipients report decreases in their pain level after a reiki session. I feel very fortunate that our hospice has a number of volunteers who have had the exacting training reiki involves, and equally grateful that I have had this training as well.

Reiki training is structured in levels, with First Degree, Second Degree, Advanced Training, and Masters levels. I have been practicing reiki for over a decade with the First and Second Degree certification. I recently met Patricia Williams, who practices and teaches Reiki in Vero Beach, Florida, and received the Advanced Training certification from her. This inspired me to repeat my earlier certifications through her as well. This experience was a wonderful lesson in the importance of finding the "right" teacher. Now a dear friend, Patricia has taught me a whole new reverence and passion for reiki, which has enhanced my practice one hundred fold.

Although, as I noted above, reiki can be done at a distance, the typical reiki session is done one-on-one. The reiki practitioner puts his or her hands on the recipient very gently, resting them outside the clothing. No manipulation or massage is done, as the technique involves energy rather than tangible or direct action. Intention and focus are key. A full reiki session would typically incorporate soothing music and involve the full body. That is rarely realistic for someone like me, whose job as a hospice nurse does not allow for lengthy treatment sessions. Instead, with a patient's permission, I would simply place my hands lightly over the site of pain or discomfort for three to five minutes. This is often enough to provide some relief.

In addition to reiki and reflexology, I often do some therapeutic touch, which works primarily with a person's energy field, or aura. Because there is no physical contact with the body, this can be a helpful option. Shirley, a 75-year-old volunteer who has been with our hospice for over seven years, tells me that she uses therapeutic touch more than any other modality. Her repertoire includes reiki, meditation, and deep lymphatic massage, to name just a few, but she finds that therapeutic touch produces the fastest, most dramatic results—not only for patients, but also for families and, in facilities, staff.

One of the things I like about complementary modalities is that because they are non-invasive and have no "side effects," they can be used together as well as individually. As a practitioner, I can use my intuition and the patient's responses to gauge what is working, and to combine a variety of methods. Needless to say, this is in stark contrast to Western medicine, which can be riskily or painfully invasive, involve difficult side effects, or be dangerous when used in certain combinations.

I recently worked with a fifty-three year old banker who benefited greatly from a combination of complementary therapies. A world traveler, Clark's situation fell between the proverbial cracks in terms of insurance, and my first visits to him were made purely as a "friend of a friend." He and his wife were initially reluctant to pay for hospice privately, as they did not know how long the process would take. After several visits during which I offered Reiki and reflexology, I could see that the timeframe for his death was closer to days or weeks than months. Clark did officially sign on to our hospice service, and died shortly thereafter.

Clark's story shows how unexpected patient reactions can be. I would have expected a sophisticated "numbers person" like Clark to feel most comfortable with linear, cognitive, analytical treatment like that of Western medicine. Typically, it is those with a more "right brain" disposition who are open to the more intuitive holistic modalities. In fact, he had had reiki treatment in the past, had responded well to it, and was completely open to holistic help now.

I first met Clark at the end of a very long and tiring day. My initial desire was just to go home rather than to make another visit. However,

I was afraid that I would not be able to get there again for many days, so I pushed on to the appointment instead. Clark had just returned from a Red Sox game, to which his son had taken him. He was very weak, weighing less than one hundred pounds. He had had a tracheotomy, so he had to write his thoughts down rather than speak them aloud. After I introduced myself, I explained exactly what I was going to do, adding a brief introduction to each modality. I told him that he should relax, and in fact that he could sleep through the session if he felt able to. His breathing deepened as I did a combination of therapeutic touch, reiki and reflexology. His wife, with whom I felt an instant connection, marveled at how peaceful he became.

When I returned several days later, Clark seemed more fidgety and restless than he had at our previous meeting. I asked him if the reflexology I was doing was too much for him. Instead, he scribbled MORE across his paper. He asked for this treatment several more times before he died. I was grateful that I had been able to take this time with him and his family. We all felt the benefit of this soulful connection, and the sense of peace and balance that resulted from it.

Hospice and the services it provides are not technically considered to be "holistic" in the sense the word is used today. I do believe hospice is holistic in the deeper sense of the word, which has to do with wholeness and connection. As hospice workers, we address the whole patient—mind, body, and spirit—and the whole family as well. Our care does not, and cannot, stop with care for the body. Death is more than simply a physical event, as the inclusion of chaplains, social workers, and therapists on the hospice team suggests.

In the past when hospice did incorporate "holistic" services, they were provided largely by volunteers, as they did not fit within the rubric of what hospice officially provided. As I noted earlier, more and more hospices are now beginning not only to use but to hire and compensate holistic nurses, massage therapists, aromatherapists, and music and art therapists. The role these additional services play can be absolutely transformative in the quality of a patient's life.

One example clearly illustrates the importance of holistic care in hospice. I remember being with the family of a dying middle-aged man many years ago. As often happens, his family struggled during the hours when death was imminent. No one wanted to leave, but no one knew what to do, either…with the best of intentions, they simply stood around uncomfortably, watching and waiting. I asked what kind of music the patient liked. I would usually suggest soft, soothing music, but that's not always the right choice. As it turned out, the patient loved…Elvis! I must say that Elvis transformed that room from a place of awkwardness, "doom" and "gloom" to one of laughter and joy. I am sure that the music and the energy it helped create were far truer to the patient than the formal silence had been, *and* far more healing for both patient and family. Elvis's music isn't what we think of when we think of music therapy, but it was surely therapeutic that blessed night.

One of the crucial steps in a peaceful death is letting go. Virtually anyone who has worked around the dying will tell you that weeping and other signs of grief, however natural they may be, can make it difficult for a patient to feel it is okay for them to depart. This is one of the reasons many patients subconsciously "orchestrate" their death at a time when family members have stepped out for even a few minutes. Some people seem to need to be alone at this time, perhaps because they sense that their loved ones will be distressed as they draw their last breath.

Sitting vigil with a dying patient can be a profoundly sacred experience, but like most hospice nurses, I usually advise families not to be overly attached to being there at the last breath. Family members often feel that not being present at that time is a sign that they did not love the patient or were not loved in return. Sometimes, the very opposite is true: they are deeply loved, to the extent that the patient does not want to distress or upset them. As always with hospice work, you have to trust in the divine plan (however you define and visualize it). If you are supposed to be there for the last breaths, you will be; if not, it was simply not what your loved one needed.

Difficult Choices: Thomas

As I hope that this book has illustrated, each and every hospice patient's situation is unique and personal. There is no typical, much less stereotypical, story. In sharing Thomas's story with you, I do not mean to suggest that it is any kind of "usual" or "average" case. Instead, it is simply a story of the difficult choices hospice patients and their families face, as well as the courage and wisdom they so often muster in response.

Thomas came into my life in early June, 2007. He was a 56-year-old former toolmaker, born in Oklahoma but living in Massachusetts at the time of our meeting. Thomas's family heritage was partially Native American. As I mentioned when speaking of Roger, I believe that this heritage—whether it is "in the blood," as it was for Thomas, or merely a passion, as it was for Roger—is one of deep spirituality, reverence, and connection. Thomas exemplified all of these things—and had, as well, a delightfully colorful and unique personality.

In March 2007, Thomas had been diagnosed with cancer of the throat. As often happens with such diagnoses, this news gave him some very difficult choices to make. According to the doctor who gave him the diagnosis, the medical treatment that would be required if he hoped to save his life was lengthy and extreme. Daily radiation would be required for many weeks, as would chemotherapy. He would need a feeding tube for some period - twenty weeks to a year. The radiation would "cook" everything in his throat. Hopefully, the tumor would be affected, but he would also lose his voice, larynx, salivary glands and taste buds. In Thomas's usual colorful way of speaking, he would end up "not knowing if I was eating a dog turd or a ribeye."

The steel rod implanted in Thomas's cervical spine as a result of an earlier medical problem was another concern. When Thomas asked what radiation treatment would do to this implant, the doctor said, "I don't know." Probably nothing, but I'm not sure." Thomas told me that he walked out of the appointment feeling less like a person than like a guinea pig.

As Thomas explained, a subsequent appointment with an oncologist felt more human and more respectful, even though the grim news did not change. "This doctor was very honest and straight-shooting with me, but also very kind," Thomas said. "He explained that chemotherapy alone was not an option; if I wanted treatment, I had to do the whole thing." This doctor also offered Thomas the option of hospice, which had never been mentioned at his meeting with the first doctor.

For Thomas, this was not a difficult decision to make. With the "six months to live" news ringing in his mind, he sped home and went straight to his calendar. Marking each square with a descending number, he ended up on November 15, 2007, the end of the six months the doctor had described.

Thomas lost no time in gathering up his son, who was sixteen at the time. They traveled for several weeks, visiting Thomas's family. Thomas also used the time to teach his son about their Native American heritage. When they returned, he scheduled the appointment at which his oncologist referred him to hospice care.

It was a sunny June morning when I first met Thomas and admitted him to our hospice service. We sat together at his kitchen table. I was immediately drawn to his matter of fact, accepting demeanor. It was so refreshing to be able to speak openly and earnestly about death and dying. I felt a close, immediate kinship with this man.

Thomas's significant other, Lisa, joined us for part of our first meeting. Thomas himself had little fear of death. Lisa was more anxious. She asked searching yet appropriate questions about how the weeks might progress, what his death would be like, and what she would be expected to do. Lisa was especially concerned that she would be alone with Thomas at the time he died. I assured her that our service would help prepare her for this possibility and, knowing that this was a concern, that we would be sure to get a nurse out very promptly. I welcomed the chance to discuss these issues in detail and answer all possible questions, as this always makes for better care.

Thomas's own questions focused on what the progression of his disease might be like. I told him the usual course would be that as the time passed he would eat less and sleep more. I explained that as the tumor grew we would likely administer medication which would decrease swelling, as well as morphine when necessary to handle pain and help with breathing. I reassured him that we would always honor his particular needs and wishes.

Once Lisa left for work, Thomas showed me some of his Native American artifacts, which were placed throughout the house. We swapped stories about Native American traditions and our experiences with them. I felt privileged to see the model planes that he built and flew as well. I can remember walking away from our two-hour admission visit feeling inspired.

I knew already that this meeting would be significant for me, just as certainly as I knew on May 2nd, 2003 that I would write this book. Naturally, it was also clear that if Thomas agreed, he would be part of the book as well.

Thomas gladly gave me permission to tell his story. We set up a meeting, which turned out to be on November 15—that is, "Day Zero" from that first marking of his calendar. It was hard to believe that nearly six months had passed since I had admitted him to our hospice service. He told me about what had happened in that time and how wonderful hospice had been in his journey. Like so many others, Thomas proclaimed that "I could never have done this without hospice."

The first time we met about telling his story, Thomas mentioned that he rarely told people he had cancer. When I asked why, he replied that "I feel dirty and I can't wash it off." He commented that a friend of his, who had also had cancer, had the same feeling. I ended our session with a relaxation exercise designed to help him visualize a divine white light coming in through the top of his head and purifying his body.

By the time we next met, Thomas had moved out of Lisa's home and was living with his son and his ex-wife (times two! they had divorced, remarried, and divorced again) of twelve years. He was there for several months, but later came to feel that he needed his independence. As was true with Thomas, a serious or terminal illness may increase the amount of care a person needs *without* decreasing the need for independence that is part of their life as an adult. No matter how complex their physical needs may be, adult patients do not become children, and always appreciate being treated with appropriate dignity and respect. Thomas felt the need to be self-reliant very strongly. He wanted to take care of himself and, ideally, die peacefully by himself, not because he did not love those closest to him but because independence was simply part of his nature and his values.

Admittedly, Thomas could sometimes take this to extremes. In fact, he actually drove his car the night before he died. This was not something any of his caregivers would have seen as safe, either for Thomas or for anyone else on the road. I am sure that no one around him gave him permission for this! Luckily, Thomas returned home without any mishaps, either to himself or to anyone else. Thomas died peacefully by himself in his apartment, as he had hoped would happen. Though Lisa found him when she visited that day, she was not present for his passing, which was the way she had hoped it would be as well.

The people who are most significant or inspirational in our lives are not always those we spend the most time with. My meetings with Thomas were relatively few, and the time span during which he was part of my life was relatively brief. Yet even at our first meeting it seemed as though we had known each other for years. There was something familiar and "real" about him that made him feel like a kindred spirit.

And, as so often happens, caregiving in Thomas's case did not all go only in one direction. I am grateful to have had the opportunity of serving him, but equally grateful for the many ways he enriched my life in return. At its best, hospice work is always a collaboration. Guided by the patient's needs and wishes, the team works together to create the best possible quality of life for whatever time is left. I will always remember Thomas: as a man who handled the ending months of his life with dignity and strength...as a friend with whom I shared both sadness and joy...and as a strong, unique, and courageous spirit.

Ten Helpful Facts About The Dying Process

1. Patients who are dying may lose interest in eating, change their food preferences and desires, and/or become physically unable to eat. Their refusal does not mean that they will starve or be in pain. These changes are a natural part of the process through which the body shuts down, and in fact the body secretes endorphins, its natural "painkillers," during the dying process. Several medications can be recommended to stimulate appetite, if and when appropriate.

2. Most (though not all) patients who know that they are dying experience some change in their spiritual attitude. Impending death often leads us to face issues we have not addressed before or inspires a new kind of curiosity. Some people return to an earlier faith. Some feel the need to make amends or otherwise come to terms with issues from their past. Some raise spiritual questions of a kind they may have shown no interest in earlier. All of these changes are normal and natural.

3. Nights can be difficult for the dying and their caregivers. The dying often suffer from changes to, or disturbances in, their sleep. Studies also show that many patients have greater fear at night than during the day. And because the patient does not sleep, the caregiver(s) may not either. Scheduling family or friends to sleep over, if possible, can help the patient as well as relieving the primary caregiver(s) during the night, resting them for the long days ahead.

4. Current research suggests that hearing is the last of the senses to go, and that a patient may be able to hear (and to some extent, take in) sounds after they seem unconscious—even after they stop breathing. Family may wish to speak to the patient right up until the end and in the minutes immediately thereafter, and/or play soft music of a kind he or she enjoyed.

5. The rate and characteristics of respiration, body temperature, physical movements, and skin coloring often change during the dying process, sometimes well before death actually occurs. The changes can seem alarming at times, but as death draws close the dying person him or herself is not usually acutely aware of them. Hospice nurses are familiar with these changes. They tell you what to expect and if what you are observing is normal. Most hospices provide written information on this as well.

6. Signs of withdrawal and lack of interest are normal, and do not mean that the patient is angry with family or friends. As a person makes their final transition, their physical and emotional connection to this world naturally shuts down. How this occurs varies from person to person and situation to situation. One patient may become sleepy or withdrawn many days before they die, while another might be able to talk, touch and engage until close to the last moment. Conversely, some patients experience a surge of energy or connection as their time approaches. They may want to talk, feel "suddenly" ready to make decisions that they have been putting off, or choose to eat after having taken no food for a time…all a part of the shifting energy and processing of the impending death experience.

7. People often improve once signed onto hospice service. Often this is a result of the tapering-off of unnecessary medications, the greater availability of care, and hospice's expertise in pain management and symptom control.

8. Unfinished business may affect the comfort and ease with which a person dies. Those with a sense of things undone sometimes linger, while those with a feeling of closure may depart with greater ease. A fear of death can also delay the process. The difference is not usually one of conscious choice, but rather a sub- or unconscious one.

9. Though those closest to a dying person often want to be there at the end, this is not always the wish of the patient. A dying person may be afraid to distress their loved one or simply prefer, consciously or unconsciously, to make their passage on their own. This is not a sign of any lack of love or regard, nor is it something a family member should ever feel guilty about. Sometimes it is just too difficult for the dying person to leave their loved one. I personally believe that this, like everything else, happens as it should, and that we should trust the divine process.

10. Though many patients and their loved ones dread the moment of death, many of my patients' families report that it is actually a moment of great joy. Many—even those who are not spiritually or religiously inclined—say that the sense of release, passage, and freedom is palpable and that the moment can be very beautiful.

Part Three: The Why, Who, Where and When of Hospice

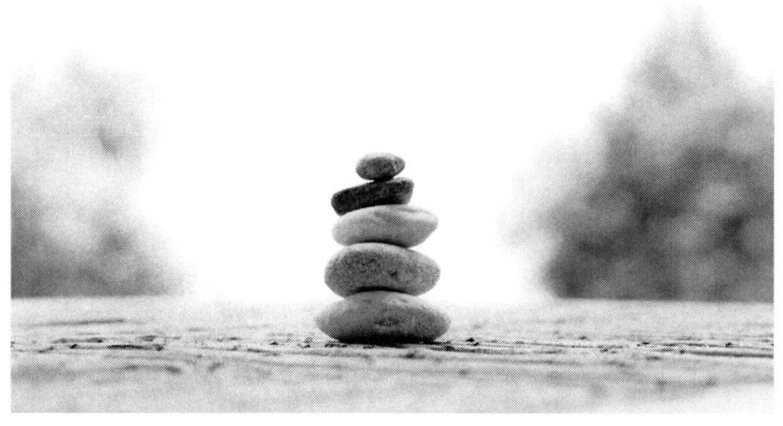

I call upon you from the ends of the earth
with heaviness in my heart; set me upon the rock
that is higher than I.

—Psalm 61

Life, Death and Hospice

When I admit a patient to our service, I almost always start out by asking them what they know about hospice. Many if not most people do not know much. Still more have misconceptions. It's not uncommon for patients to respond to a suggestion of hospice help with something like "Oh, no, I'm not ready for *that*." Some of the motivation for such responses comes from denial about the reality and imminence of death. But statements like that also arise from a misunderstanding of what hospice is, does, and means.

It is true that hospice work begins when a patient receives the diagnosis of a life-threatening illness. Usually, the patient is referred when a doctor estimates that if the individual's present condition progresses at its normal anticipated rate, the patient will have six months or less to live. This specific benchmark may change over time, as medical guidelines are becoming more and more stringent.

Yet as I've spoken about earlier, this timeframe is rarely hard-and-fast. Medicine is far from infallible, even in the hands of excellent providers. Prognoses are proven wrong virtually every day. In addition, the enhanced care a patient receives from hospice can actually help him or her live considerably longer than has been estimated. Statistics show that the extra care, combined with pain- and symptom-control methods, can stabilize a patient's condition. The patient may be decertified from hospice care, and be certified and decertified as many times as necessary. Happily, there is no limit to how often an individual patient may be signed on to hospice care. Conversely, knowing that they and their family are safe, some patients may actually die earlier than expected.

For all of these reasons, no competent hospice provider would ever take a patient's hope away. As I have said before, miracles happen every day, and those of us who work in a hospice capacity see them far more often than others might expect.

Some of the misconceptions people have about hospice come from the fact that it works differently from the way everyday medicine does. In some ways, hospice may do less than "ordinary" medicine. Painful or debilitating treatments are typically not provided, for example; comfort, rather than cure, is the goal, and all or virtually all intrusive testing and treatments are stopped. In addition, a patient who has been hospitalized may be moved home if sufficient resources of space, caregivers, and a safe environment are available to provide the care that is necessary in conjunction with hospice help, allowing the patient the greater privacy and dignity of dying at home.

In other ways, hospice sometimes offers *more* services than is typical of "normal" medical care. For example, while hospice does not provide care "24/7," we are on call to answer questions or help with emergencies. Visits to doctors' offices are no longer required once a patient cannot make the trip easily; instead, in-home care is provided by doctors or, in many situations, by the nurses who work closely with them. Hospice serves not only the patient but also their family, helping them understand the dying process and deal with their own emotions as well as teaching them to give physical care. Similarly, hospice care includes not just attention to physical symptoms but also emotional needs. As this suggests, hospice work takes for granted that patients are not just individual physical bodies, but persons with physical, emotional and spiritual needs as well as deep connections to families and friends that are also affected by the diagnosis.

I have said often that hospice is not a death sentence. With the stories above in mind you can see why it can almost be called a *life* sentence. That is, from the moment a patient is signed up with hospice, quality of life is the goal and criteria. Where medical treatment often abandons quality of life in order to extend *length* of life—even when the time gained is minimal and spent in discomfort or pain—hospice is concerned to provide quality of life regardless of the timeframe. The difference does not sound huge but, in truth, it is.

Where the first two sections of this book was focused on personal stories, this section talks about some of the more logistical aspects of hospice. As always, my intent here is not to provide an encyclopedic treatment of the subject. Instead, my purpose is simply to help demystify hospice, its team, and its services. By describing each of these aspects more fully from the personal viewpoint of a longtime hospice provider, I hope to help dispel some of the fear-based myths that surround hospice, and to inspire at least some readers to embrace rather than shun this extraordinary resource.

The History of Hospice

Cultures throughout history have always developed their own special ways of caring for the dying. Our own word "hospice" comes from the Latin *hospes*, a term that could mean either "host" or "guest." The first hospices were the monasteries located along the European pilgrimage routes, where pilgrims going to the Holy Land, Santiago de Compostela in Spain, or other holy sites would stop for food and lodging. Monasteries served as both guesthouses for travelers and also as hospitals during this time—and because so many pilgrims were people seeking cure for an intractable illness, the monasteries along the pilgrimage routes cared for more than their share of seriously ill and dying patients. For that matter, even the healthiest of those walking thousands of miles on pilgrimage surely needed the nurturance the monasteries could provide!

Strange as it seems to those of us living in modern times, dying did not come to be looked at primarily as a medical event until the 19th century. Until then, relatively few serious illnesses were actually curable, while trained doctors were in relatively short supply outside of urban centers. Instead of being treated by the medical establishment, the dying were largely cared for by their families, their communities, or their churches, and death was seen mostly as a spiritual and personal, rather than medical, milestone. However, a scattering of facilities similar to modern hospices did exist in France, Ireland, and England by the turn of the twentieth century. All, I was interested to learn through my reading, were founded and run by women, most of them with either a religious or a nursing background.

Gradually, developments in medical care and technology in the nineteenth and twentieth centuries "medicalized" death, bringing it out of the hands of families and churches and into medical settings. By the mid-twentieth century, over 80% of Americans died in hospitals. Undoubtedly, new treatments, tests and drugs made it possible to live longer, and stronger, than ever before. But these same advancements also created a host of troubling problems. How much choice should patients themselves have about the manner of their own death? What is the role of doctors when a cure is no longer possible? Is life-sustaining treatment always necessary? Which is more important, preserving life or preserving quality of life? How well do doctors—who are trained to practice narrow specialties--work together to care for a dying person? How can the special pain management needs of the dying best be handled? And what about the families of terminal patients, so often left to shoulder the burden of care without emotional or social support? There was no simple answer to any of these questions, just a growing need to respond to them thoughtfully.

In response to these and other similar issues, in 1967 Dr. Cicely Saunders founded the first hospice, which included both at-home and inpatient care for the terminally ill. (The hospice, called St. Christopher's, still operates in suburban London to this day). The practices and philosophies at St. Christopher's were radical for their time, especially the focus on quality rather than length of life and the emphasis on making home, or home-like, care available to the dying whenever possible.

Later made a Dame of the British Empire, Cicely Saunders is an example of the way that extraordinary healers sometimes appear in the right place, at the right time, with just the right training and temperament. She was trained as both a social worker and a physician. Her early medical work included studying pain management for cancer patients. With this hands-on experience under her belt, she pioneered the practice of giving painkillers to dying patients on a regular schedule, rather than forcing them to wait for the pain to return, as was the norm for non-terminal patients. She also advocated multi-disciplinary care that included not just medical treatment for the dying person's body, but also emotional, spiritual, and psychological support for both patients and families. Dr. Saunders once said that "We do not need to cure to heal," a beautiful and simple statement that sums up the philosophy of hospice perfectly.

From 1968 on, a number of hospice and palliative care programs opened in England, following the St. Christopher's model. Dr. Saunders introduced the idea to America in a lecture on holistic health care given at Yale University in 1963. She continued to spread her ideas and information about hospice to medical students, chaplains, social workers and nurses as a visiting faculty member at Yale in 1965. Florence Wald, then the Director of the Yale School of Nursing, supported Saunders' work in this country, even taking a sabbatical to study hospice at St. Christopher's before continuing to spread the word back in America. Just like so many holistic philosophies did later on, the concepts of hospice spread through an informal network of passionate advocates, each passing on new ideas and information to those with whom they worked.

The history of hospice can't be accurately told without also mentioning Dr. Elisabeth Kübler-Ross, who helped bring the concept to America and changed the way our culture looks at dying. Born and raised in Switzerland, Dr. Kübler-Ross experienced the deaths of loved ones in her early life and the widespread pain of World War II, during which she worked with refugees in Poland. Coming to America in 1957 and earning her credentials as a psychiatrist here, she was a firm believer in the connection of body and mind—not a conviction that was the norm among doctors at the time!—and a passionate advocate for the right of all patients, whatever their situation, to be treated with dignity and respect.

Her 1969 book, *On Death and Dying*, was based on more than five hundred interviews with terminal patients. Viewing dying as just one more stage of life, giving the dying a voice and allowing them to speak to a broad audience for what was really the first time, the book became a huge bestseller despite the fact that discussions of death and dying were still socially avoided. The impact of this ground-breaking book on the brand-new hospice movement, and on the treatment of the terminally ill generally, can't be over-emphasized. It introduced so many valuable facts and concepts about the dying experience that we take for granted today.

Dr. Kübler-Ross famously identified the five stages of the dying experience, stages that are also undergone by those in grief. She approached dying persons as people with spiritual and emotional as well as physical needs, rather than seeing them as impersonal "patients" or "cases" as traditional medicine tended to do. Her book advocates giving dying patients choice about their care; listening to the wisdom they have to share; and offering patients the option for care and death at home, rather than only institutional treatment.

In her testimony at the first national hearings on dying with dignity, given by the United States Senate Special Committee on Aging in 1972, Kübler-Ross stated, "We isolate both the dying and the old, and it serves a purpose. They are reminders of our own mortality. We should not institutionalize people. We can give families…the spiritual, emotional and financial help in order to facilitate the final care at home." In the late 1970s, Kübler-Ross founded her own hospice and hospice training facilities, first in California and then in Virginia. She worked tirelessly for the cause of holistic medicine and wrote nineteen books in addition to *On Death and Dying*. This extraordinary woman died in 2004, but her work lives vibrantly on.

The first American hospice was opened in Connecticut in 1974, serving those with cancer, ALS, and a variety of other terminal conditions. By the late 1970s, hospice was beginning to be recognized as a viable alternative for the care of the terminally ill in America, and hospice demonstration projects were being offered across the country by the Health Care Financing Administration. Medicare coverage for hospice care was introduced in the early 1980s and signed into permanent law in 1986. From the government's point of view at least, hospice had "arrived," though much still needed to be done to assure its growth as a widely available and accurately understood alternative.

The beginnings of the AIDS epidemic in the 1980s brought new and broader awareness of issues related to death and dying. At that time, AIDS was usually fatal from one or more of a variety of complications. It was widely, sometimes cruelly, misunderstood even in hospitals and medical settings. (To demonstrate just how punitively the disease was seen, when Dr. Kübler-Ross, already quite famous by then, tried to established a hospice for babies with AIDS in 1986, she was forced to abandon the idea due to widespread community resistance.) The approach to dying developed by Drs. Saunders and Kübler-Ross was needed more than ever, both in its emphasis on compassion and its focus on teamwork and effective symptom management. Tragic as they were, the first years of the AIDS epidemic, with their many thousands of deaths of comparatively young people, continued to build American awareness of how important it is to offer the dying choice, respect, and dignity—even when they are shunned by traditional medical facilities.

Statistics from 2008, the latest year for which full numbers are available as I write this, show how far American hospice has come in its thirty-odd years. There were 3,257 Medicare-certified hospices in the U.S. that year, serving more than a million patients annually, along with another few hundred volunteer-based organizations that were not Medicare certified. About two thousand of the hospices were dedicated hospice agencies, with the remainder being nursing home, hospital, or home health agency-based. Approximately fifteen percent of hospices offered residential treatment, averaging at around thirteen beds each. Hospice use by minorities was growing slowly but steadily, as was hospice care for patients with a diagnosis of a non-cancer condition. Paid staff positions in hospice were growing, but volunteers remained key providers of services. In 2007, the last year in which statistics on that particular issue are available, a total of more than 88,000 paid employees (including all of the members of the hospice team I describe elsewhere in this book) work for hospice, while a total of almost 48,000 serve on a volunteer basis.

Hospice care is now available in some form in over forty countries around the world. However, it—and good medical care generally—is far from a given, especially in less developed nations. World Health

Organization studies show that opioid drugs and skilled practitioners remain scarce, making it difficult both to find and to provide good palliative care. Whenever I feel frustrated by the many ways hospice is still misunderstood, I try to remind myself of how lucky we are as Americans to have this priceless resource available in so many communities, often at a very modest cost.

The Hospice Team

As I have noted earlier, at the heart of every hospice is the team. Recently I met with a hospice social worker I had worked with over ten years ago. We ended up reminiscing about a case we shared together in the late 1990s. This case makes a perfect introduction to my discussion of the hospice team. It suggests not only how many "hats" each of us wear, but also how willing the various members are to pitch in to help in special situations.

At the time I met him, Stan was a man in his late thirties. He had liver cancer and, with it, uncontrolled pain. At his admission meeting, Stan was asked what his goal from our service was, a question we always ask. His answer was that he wanted "to see my 3-year-old son, Joey, turn 4." Joey's birthday turned out to be the day before Christmas. At the time, Christmas was still over a month away and it seemed most unlikely that Stan would be alive that long. When I brought this story to our interdisciplinary team meeting the following day, their reaction was astonishing and immediate. "If Stan won't make it until Christmas, then we will have Christmas—and his son's birthday—early!"

With his wife's delighted blessings, the team swung into action. The social worker met with the family to see what special needs, wishes and wants they had. Stan asked if someone would get his wife a red teddy as a gift from him. Immediately, my colleague and friend went out and bought a huge red teddy bear...only to feel totally embarrassed when the social worker showed up with a red *lingerie* teddy. I guess this just goes to show that even when everyone is working together efficiently and with the best of intentions, confusions can occur. Our Home Health Aides began baking, our pastoral counselor went out and rented a Santa suit, and a male volunteer went to cut down a Christmas tree, which he delivered to Stan's home and decorated with the family. The entire staff helped get Christmas gifts and donations from varied community resources. Within three days, our team had created a really incredible Christmas.

The moment when "Santa" walked through the door with a huge bag of toys and gifts was an amazing one. Joey hid under the kitchen table at first, clearly overwhelmed with astonishment. Once the presents started to go under the tree, he quickly mustered up the courage to see what goodies Santa had brought him. I acted as Santa's helper that day, organizing the food the team members had prepared and taking pictures of the festivities. I got plenty of shots of Stan and his wife together, as well as of Joey opening his gifts. Stan and his wife at once laughed and cried as they watched him open present after present, representing both birthday and Christmas. Santa, Joey and I ate cookies in the kitchen while Stan and his wife took some private time to open the teddy and their other gifts.

Stan died several days later. Our entire staff attended the wake. At the service, Stan's wife shared that she had spent his last night with him in his hospital bed…wearing his Christmas gift to her. There, in the casket with him, lay that same red teddy. For the record, that teddy was the lingerie, not the teddy bear.

So indeed, hospice is a team. No one type of caregiver could possibly provide hospice's wide range of services. This is even true of its medical directors and doctors. In everyday medicine, doctors are at the top of the status pyramid. Nurses, therapists, aides, social workers and so on are assumed to serve less critical roles. Hospice approaches this rather differently. Because a cure is no longer sought and the diagnosis has already been made at the time a patient is signed on to hospice service, the M.D.'s expertise is not as central as it would otherwise be considered, and a variety of other providers often offer the most crucial care.

I don't say this to suggest that doctors are not important to hospice. On the contrary. A doctor's special expertise in diagnosis, pain management, medications and dosages, symptom control, and so on are, of course, very important. I only want to emphasize that *everyone* working at and for hospice plays a crucial role. A home health aide or volunteer can mean just as much to the patient's quality of life and the family's comfort as a far more "important" provider. The hospice team uses, values, and appreciates the special gifts and skills of each and every one of its different members.

The makeup and roles of this team may vary somewhat from hospice to hospice, depending on issues such as budget, size of patient load or geographic region covered, and whether or not the hospice works with hospitals and/or has its own hospice facility. Whatever the differences from one hospice to the next, I can say with some confidence that virtually every hospice team is both very diverse and very busy. Each hospice provides many patients in many locations with many different services, on many different timetables and with many different and unique considerations along the way. That's a lot of "manys," but I use them to emphasize just how many variables there are in the care any hospice gives.

Integrating all of these different services and coordinating the efforts of myriad hospice workers is therefore a real challenge! In my own experience I find that I might overlap with one volunteer frequently for a time then rarely see him or her again; similarly, I might almost never see other nurses, our chaplain, or other team members in person. Phone calls, voicemails, email—all of these are key methods we use to communicate and collaborate. But our key strategy in this regard is regular interdisciplinary team meetings. At my hospice, these sessions are held by each team every two weeks. Virtually all of the team members come together for these sessions, which can therefore involve as many as twenty or thirty participants sitting together at once. The meetings take place in our conference room and typically last about two to three hours. The volunteer coordinator attends and volunteers may join us as well, but they are not required to do so.

The heart of the meeting is the review of each and every case currently on our service. Our medical director, an M.D., is present to consult on medical concerns. In addition, caregiving challenges, family issues and conflicts, and any other questions are discussed and resolved, with each team member involved reporting on his or her experiences with the patient. This dialogue allows us to learn from each other's experiences, come up with good strategies, and provide the most seamlessly coordinated care possible.

With that said, let me share some perspectives on the individual members of the hospice team.

Medical directors. The medical director is an M.D. who supervises the medical aspects of each hospice case. In some larger hospices he or she may oversee other doctors as well. In my hospice, the medical director covers patients who do not have their own primary doctor; in other hospice organizations, the hospice medical director becomes *every* patient's primary doctor at the time the patient is signed on to hospice service. As always, the details may differ, but the intent is the same: comprehensive, coordinated care under the guidance of a medical professional who is expert in hospice issues.

Hospice nurses. I have already talked at length about my experiences as a hospice nurse. What is missing from this hands-on, personal picture is a glimpse of the administrative, organizational and technical work that goes on behind the scenes of hospice nursing. Without both of these halves, the picture is not complete.

It will be no surprise when I say that hospice nursing is very complicated, involving many staffers and many forms of treatment as well, of course, as many patients. Keeping this complex, interconnected system of care going, and going well, is quite the task. The nature of our job means that we nurses spend much of our working time with patients or on the road between them. If we did not have strong routines, thoughtful systems, and careful checks and balances behind us, our work could not be effective.

Before I begin this description, I want to note that this picture of how the hospice nurse and team work is based on my own experience and my own particular hospice. While the same basic principles apply across the board, each hospice has its own particular systems, which vary with its size, its geographical "reach," its staffing, its affiliations and so on. The details I share here may not be the same ones experienced by nurses or patients from other hospices. Instead, this explanation of hospice nursing from a more technical point of view is simply meant to give the general reader a sense of how the practicalities function, and also to evoke how much scrupulously precise administrative effort goes on behind the hospice nurse patients meet face to face.

Because mine is a large hospice, serving anywhere from about 150 to 200 patients at a time, our nurses are organized using three shifts: one from 4:00 p.m. to 12:00 a.m., one from 12:00 a.m. to 8:00 a.m., and one from 8:00 a.m. to 4:00 p.m. (In a smaller hospice, on-call times rather than actual working shifts might rotate.) Because nurses are assigned to every shift, someone is on call around the clock. When I admit a patient to our hospice service, I always assure the families that if they have a question in the middle of the night, they do not need to hesitate before calling, as the nurse who will answer their phone call is not one who has already worked all day and trying to get some sleep.

The hospice I serve covers a fairly large region, so its nurses are organized in geographical teams. Each nurse carries a caseload of somewhere between eight and fifteen patients, for whom he or she is the primary nurse. The primary is the nurse who is officially assigned that patient, usually right at the time of admission. Primary assignments are made based on a number of factors including geographical location and, sometimes, language. We are fortunate enough to have a Spanish-speaking nurse, and of course she is the first choice for patients with Spanish as their first language. By assigning a primary nurse, we can keep the patient's care as consistent as possible. Both patients and families appreciate seeing the same face rather than a new one, as well as avoiding the necessity of asking their questions or explaining their situation to a series of people.

We all gather on Monday morning for team meeting, followed by staff meeting for nurses only. Our gatherings begin with a candle-lit moment of silence, followed by a reading of the list of patients who have died during the week. Everyone is given the chance to talk about these patients, and to share with the others how each passing went. This time of sharing allows each of us to process our loss, and to learn from the experience of our peers.

Once this meeting is over, everyone scatters to their desks. (We nurses don't spend much time at our hospice offices, but we each have a small desk/cubicle where we can make phone calls, store items, meet with other staff, and so on.) Our first job is to call each and every patient our team is currently serving to assess who needs to be seen, and when. This is a triage process, just like that used in an emergency room, and its purpose is the same, to prioritize time and resources.

Generally, we set up appointments at the beginning of each week, confirming right before each visit to make sure that the time still works for the patient and/or family. It's routine to see each patient once a week unless something makes more frequent visits necessary. Dressings might need to be changed daily, for example, or the patient's symptoms might have become more pronounced as he or she grew closer to death. These same kinds of factors mean that our schedules are constantly subject to changes and additions. On weekdays when we as nurses are either on the road doing appointments or off duty, we have a supervisor to triage calls, making sure that each of us knows when a patient has urgent needs or their loved ones have urgent questions. We are always available to assist.

The first meeting any of us have with a patient is the so-called informational visit, which I have mentioned before. This meeting, which like all of our services is free of charge, occurs to discuss options and share information with the patient and/or family. The patient may or may not be signed on to hospice service at this time. When admission is desired and appropriate, a separate visit for that purpose is made.

The admission visit may take anywhere from one to three hours depending on the circumstances. People usually have many concerns, and the admitting nurse takes the time to answer all questions and do some teaching about how hospice works. We have usually been brought into the picture because the patient has been told there is nothing more that can be done in their case. The natural response is shock, fear, and uncertainty. When I first arrive at a home on the admission visit, I can usually feel the tension in the room the moment I walk in the door.

I usually begin admission visits by asking the people present what they know about hospice. This way, I can correct any misconceptions and banish any sense of stigma right up front. I explain that our focus is on quality of life rather than attempting any "cure," and that now that the patient has been signed on to our service, they will usually never have to go to the hospital; suffer through major tests such as MRIs, CT scans, or PET scans; or call 911. Instead, they can call hospice and a nurse will either talk them through whatever is going on, or come and make a visit. I describe the hospice team and discuss what kinds of visits and services they can expect. I emphasize that we are on call 24/7, that there is no cost for our service, and that we are there not just for the person with the life-threatening illness, but also for the entire family. As I share this information, there is almost always a subtle yet palpable shift in the energy of the room, which moves from fear and dread to a sense of relief.

With all of this introductory information out of the way, I turn the conversation to the patient. I get a short history of their present illness and any other elements of their medical history that are helpful in their care. We discuss any equipment they may need, which might include a hospital bed, specialty mattress (designed for those with skin breakdown), a wheelchair, a shower chair, a walker, or an oxygen machine. Most families are both surprised and impressed at how quickly the necessary equipment arrives—usually, within an hour or two of the admission visit. Oxygen is often particularly appreciated. Typically, people not on hospice must have an oxygen saturation of 88 or less to qualify for this equipment; once on hospice, oxygen is available without any such criteria.

Once we establish what equipment is needed, I ask if they wish to continue to visit their doctor. If they wish to and are able, they have our blessing. If not, I reassure them that there is no need to do so. Hospice nurses will be visiting, monitoring their situation, and working closely with doctors who trust our observations and expertise. In many cases, both patient and family are relieved to discover they need no longer struggle to make tiring trips to medical offices in order to obtain care.

At this point, I also get a list of all of the medications the patient is currently taking. Now that they are on our service, hospice will pay for any medications pertaining to the illness that brought them to us. (The patient continues to be responsible for any medications that have been prescribed for other, unrelated conditions.) We reconcile all medications with the attending physician, usually the oncologist if the patient has cancer; sometimes, with the approval of the doctor and the permission of patient and family, we will change one or more medications to those our pharmacy more commonly uses.

Fear of discomfort and pain is often on the minds of both the patient and the family. I am always glad to tell them that they will receive what our hospice calls a "comfort kit" the day following their admission to hospice. The kit contains a variety of medications to relieve common symptoms that may occur, including nausea, vomiting, anxiety, shortness of breath, tracheal secretions, fever, and pain. These medications may never be needed. But whatever happens, just having the kit on hand means that a patient will not need to wait for a nurse to call or a prescription to arrive if they find themselves in discomfort.

With regard to patient comfort, I also discuss morphine and its use for hospice patients at the admission visit. People in our culture often associate morphine with imminent death or fear it as a source of destructive addiction. The admission visit gives me the opportunity to banish this stigma. Many of those I admit to our service are surprised to know that morphine is useful not only in pain management but also in oxygenating the blood, which it does by lowering the respiratory threshold and causing fewer yet deeper breaths. In addition, they are usually reassured to know that being prescribed morphine is not a sign that death is around the corner. I reassure them that it is legitimately and effectively used by many people whose illnesses are not even terminal. "Make friends with the morphine" is a saying I often repeat.

Signing the necessary paperwork is, of course, part of the admission visit. Among the documents is health care proxy. This simple form names the person who the patient wishes to make medical decisions on their behalf if they were no longer able to do so. The patient may already have created a health care proxy before they are admitted to our service, and either way, the form may never be needed. But if the patient does become too incapacitated to speak for him- or herself, it is worth its weight in gold in avoiding the distressing, ugly, and costly disputes that can arise in situations where the patient's wishes are not clear and no one has the legal authority to speak on their behalf.

Another crucial document is the Do Not Resuscitate order (DNR). In the majority of cases, a DNR has already been discussed prior to a patient's admission to hospice. But knowing that some patients have either not yet been introduced to this form or not yet decided about it, I bring as much respect, compassion, and gentleness as I can to the topic. It is a touchy subject, and one that a family may need to consider and discuss before the right decision can be made.

As I note in one of this book's sidebars, signing a DNR is not required to come onto hospice service; while we believe they are helpful, we always respect the patient's wishes. My job as admission nurse is to give them the information they need to make an informed decision. For example, it is important that they know that they can always destroy a DNR if they change their mind after they sign it, and also that if no signed DNR is available, Emergency Medical Technicians are legally required to perform CPR if they are on site when the patient's breathing stops. I have found that the best way to convey the essence of the DNR is to ask the patient to decide whether, if they stopped breathing, they would wish to have CPR performed. If they would not, a DNR is appropriate.

I end the admission visit with a short physical assessment. It includes most of the tests and observations that are repeated at later visits and which I describe below.

By the end of this long visit the patient and family usually feel far more peaceful than they did at its beginning. Often, I am given a warm embrace when I depart. I always leave hoping that I will see the patient and family again, but that is only rarely possible. Even so, I almost always walk away from an admission meeting with a sense of accomplishment, grace, and a deep love for my job.

The "average" nursing visit once a patient is admitted, if there is any such thing, lasts anywhere from fifteen minutes to two or three hours. It all depends on what is going on. Each visit typically begins with a physical assessment. We will check blood pressure, pulse, color, lung sounds, edema (swelling) levels, bowel sounds, respiratory rate, temperature, and, if necessary, oxygen levels. Equally important, we will ask questions that help us assess the patient's situation, needs, and comfort. How is their pain level? How often have they moved their bowels? Are they having nausea or vomiting…tracheal secretions… urinary incontinence or retention…restlessness… shortness of breath… or other symptoms? How is their appetite?

On one visit, no changes might be needed to a patient's care or medication. On another, a variety of adjustments might be required. For example, if the patient can't control their urine or, alternatively can't urinate at all, we might need to insert a catheter so that urine is automatically drained into a collection bag. Similarly, if a patient is no longer breathing easily, I might also turn on a fan whose air will touch a patient's cheeks, a small change that can help stimulate breathing with remarkable effectiveness. Like most hospice nurses, I always want to begin with the least invasive solution possible.

Naturally, medication management is a crucial part of our jobs as hospice nurses. Each patient's primary nurse is responsible for making sure that he or she has sufficient supply for the week, if necessary re-ordering any or all of the medications covered by hospice. If a patient has new symptoms or increased pain, we contact the hospice doctor and make recommendations for treatment. The hospice pharmacy is then called, and the medicines are either ordered and delivered, or arranged through a local pharmacy.

Though they are not always needed, pain medicines are obviously a crucial part of the hospice medication picture. We always want to keep pain as well managed as possible. Our first choice in this regard is medication that can be taken orally. If that no longer works—for example, if a patient becomes unable to swallow or pills no longer control the pain well—we turn to other options.

Where necessary, pumps are available to deliver narcotics subcutaneously. These may sound "creepy" to a lay person, but are actually less invasive and more effective than intravenous injection. As a nurse I would get the pump started and then, as always, work closely with the doctor to monitor the medication, making sure that the dosage is adequate to control the pain. The patient's primary nurse is then responsible for making sure the medication being pumped does not run out, the insertion site is changed regularly, and the needle itself is changed every three days as well.

So far, all of the issues I've mentioned that I cover on a visit have been physical ones, but as was demonstrated by my earlier stories, these "nuts and bolts" services are far from the only ones rendered by hospice nurses! In the midst of checking symptoms, calling doctors, and so on, we nurses are also present to answer patient and family questions, teach loved ones skills or strategies that will help them make things more comfortable, refer them to resources, and so on. If the patient is in a nursing home or skilled facility, we consult with facility staff and also make sure to call the family member who is our primary contact as well. A multitude of issues might come up with any given "participant" on any given day.

Charting, the medical profession's special name for detailed patient record-keeping, is a fact of life for every nurse and doctor. Most people of my age got our first picture of charts as the clipboards hung at the ends of hospital beds on medical television shows. Today, however, most charting is done by computer, and my hospice is no exception. As nurses, we are supplied with dedicated laptops to ensure that strong security measures stay in place, confidentiality is complete, and everyone uses the same system. The laptops, which are networked, also allow each and every hospice team member to access up to date information on every case from wherever they may be, allowing our care to be seamless even in, say, emergencies where a nurse is suddenly unavailable.

It's a good thing that the laptops are portable, because we as nurses might use them in a variety of locations: at the patient's home during a visit, back at the hospice office, or at home. I personally do most of my charting at home, after hours. Timeliness is important in charting. New admission, for example, must be charted within forty-eight hours.

Charting is a time-consuming process because everything must be entered, from vital signs to medication changes and more. For example, we would record it if we co-facilitated a family meeting with a social worker or did a nursing supervision for a Home Health Aide. I find that I can complete my charting in fifteen minutes or so for some visits, but not by any means for all. An admission visit might take as much as two to three hours to chart, as every single fact and indication is being entered for the first time.

Like many nurses, I would have to confess that charting is not my favorite part of the job. I am a nurse because I love to work with patients, not computers. Plus, facing a pile of charting after a long day in the field can feel very daunting. But even if we don't enjoy it much, all good nurses agree that charting is crucial to good hospice care.

For obvious reasons, hospice nurses do need some time off! Physical exhaustion and emotional burnout are always possibilities. Happily, most hospice nurses work in cohesive and supportive teams. If a nurse in my hospice is overwhelmed by a particular case or by personal concerns, for example, we are all there to back him or her up in whatever way is helpful, from switching cases to switching days.

Hospice social workers. Many lay people are not aware of the important work social workers do in hospice. In my hospice, specially trained medical social workers typically visit clients one or two times a month and/or as needed. They offer a wealth of information about community resources, financial planning, family meetings, and much, much more. In addition to serving the patient him- or herself, they assist the patient's family as they deal with challenging end of life issues. They can provide a sounding board, help with conflict resolution, facilitate family meetings, and offer many other forms of support and teaching. The knowledge and skills necessary to care for a hospice patient are not "built in" to patients or their families. Like everything else, they must be learned and developed—and hospice social workers play a key role in this process.

A hospice social worker who was a colleague of mine a decade or so ago shared a funny story. "It was my very first hospice case," she told me, smiling. "I remember thinking 'what have I got myself into?' The patient was an older woman who had two daughters. When I arrived she was looking out the window at the clouds. She said that the clouds looked like a staircase…and then, the next thing I knew, she exclaimed 'There's Dad!"—and with a smile on her face, she died right then and there! It was the most heart-warming initiation into Hospice I could have had." I am sure it was also one of the simplest cases she ever had, most of our patients not leaving us quite this quickly.

David, one of our most effective social workers, said to me once that "Social workers do a considerable amount of work with hospice staff because the veil between our patients and their families, and ourselves, is very thin." We all have our own family histories and dynamics, which can get enmeshed with those of our patients and their families. Our hospice social workers are always available to help us sort through these issues.

Mary, another one of our gifted social workers, shared a story about one of her most profound cases with me as I was writing this book. Her patient was a musician in his forties who had a drug addiction, coupled with a life-threatening illness. Mary's own son was about the same age as her patient, and struggled with some similar issues. Mary recalled the many hours she spent talking with this patient about the mysteries of life, death, and the human journey. He looked at the meaning of his life with new depth during this time. He also came to know his mother—his primary caregiver—in entirely new ways, becoming more close to her than he ever had before. Mary found their process extraordinarily moving, but also had to take care to keep her strong emotional identification with mother and son from blurring the lines between her life and theirs. Her colleagues were there to support her throughout, and our monthly staff support groups proved to be a very valuable form of support as well.

Home Health Aides (HHAs). Among our most valuable team members are our Home Health Aides, or HHAs. We nurses depend on them to help keep our patients comfortable and their families supported and sane! They are our "eyes and ears," much in the same way we as nurses are the doctors' eyes and ears, providing information even when we are not there to gather it ourselves. . In every community and on every hospice service, HHAs give of themselves with generosity, grace, and skill. Given how low their wages are relative to many other hospice staff their work is truly a labor of love. In the work of people like Marilyn, the HHA whose stories I am about to share, it comes straight from respect, generosity, compassion, and a deep commitment to making a dying person's journey more bearable, more complete, more meaningful, more individual, more human, more dignified, and more holy.

HHAs handle personal care for our patients. This work varies somewhat from case to case but might encompass such tasks as bathing, shaving, changing linens, assistance with bedpans, and feeding. A HHA might prepare a quick meal, fill ice bags, do some light housekeeping, handle a load of laundry, or bring in mail from the mailbox. In ordinary life these tasks are not considered very important, but when there is a dying patient in the house things are entirely different. Some hospice patients are entirely on their own, while others are cared for by loved ones who are already overwhelmed, both emotionally and logistically. In these situations, something as "small" as adjusting a thermostat, replacing a burned-out light bulb or wiping down a patient's forehead can make all the difference.

The kinds of work HHAs do gives them the chance to really get to know patients and their families in ways that we nurses are sometimes unable to match thanks to the tight timeframes under which we work. It's not surprising that many HHAs form close bonds with the families they serve, and remain in touch with them many weeks, months or even years after a patient has died.

I'm sad to have to say that as Medicare continues to tighten regulations, HHA service time has become more limited. As of this writing, only one hour per visit is reimbursable. Under extreme circumstances this hour can be provided twice a day, but we generally start with scheduling a visit two or three days a week. The good news is that HHAs can accomplish a tremendous amount in even these short amounts of time thanks to the wealth of knowledge and experience most bring to their jobs.

Marilyn is in her fifties and is strong of body, voice, and opinions. As she herself would say, not without pride, she is a tough cookie. She has been an aide for thirty years, eight of which she has spent on hospice service. Her work illustrates the crucial and varied role aides play. When I met with her recently, stories flooded forth like water over an overflowing dam. We laughed and we cried as we shared them for almost three hours. I have always known what an amazing service

HHAs provide, but after visiting with Marilyn I was even more filled with awe and respect. What extraordinary things this one person had achieved, and how many families have reason to be deeply grateful to her.

Marilyn would never boast, but the stories she shared with me made clear how far out of her way, and beyond the confines of her job, she went for the good of her patients. One example was a case in which the patient was a 42-year-old mom with two young boys and a rapidly-growing cancer. The patient's husband was a sophisticated man and the patient's job was conservative as well—but the patient herself had always leaned toward colorful, bohemian styles, and actually had once wanted to live the life of a hippie! This long-buried dream came back as she spoke to Marilyn during her last weeks. Together, they came up with a plan. Marilyn brought in her own VCR, bought her scarves and jewelry, and helped her dress in fun hippie garb. Together, they taped videotapes for the patient to leave for her children and husband. Each family member got an eight-hour tape for all of those special occasions that the patient would miss, from birthdays and graduations to weddings and the births of grandchildren. Marilyn even videotaped the patient reading many children's books to the grandchildren she would never meet.

The final story Marilyn told me on that day touched my heart just as much. It concerned an elderly gentleman who had been in her care for approximately six months. Finally his wife of fifty years could no longer care for him, and he was admitted to the VA Hospital. Upon admission, he kept asking for his girlfriend. The VA staff politely assured him that his wife was right there. Yet he continued to call out for this "other woman."

The patient's wife had called Marilyn, to whom they had grown close over the months, and let her know that he was close to dying. When Marilyn arrived at the facility—on her own time, of course—the nurses explained the odd situation and asked her if she had any suggestions as to what to do. Marilyn sheepishly confessed to them that she was the girlfriend—though only in a playful sense of the word.

Marilyn knew that her male patients still needed to feel like men, not like mere withering bodies consumed by illness, weakness and decay. A silly endearment or two—with the spouse's knowledge and approval, of course!—helped make this patient laugh and feel more whole. To my mind, this unusual bit of assistance was just as valuable as the actual tasks Marilyn had done for the couple.

Indeed, the patient's wife was the first to welcome Marilyn to the hospital bedside and tell her husband that his "girlfriend" had arrived. As Marilyn kissed him on the cheek, he smiled. Within a few minutes, with his wife holding one hand and this special "girlfriend" holding the other, he died peacefully. Three years later, Marilyn and the patient's wife still keep in touch.

This story is not just an example of the unique role of the HHA, but also a reminder of how the hospice team can truly become part of a family—right at the time the family needs love, understanding, and support the most. Sometimes there are just no words to describe the sacred bonds that are developed. A special grace is bestowed that helps heal the grieving hearts of the families as well as our own. This is what makes us love our jobs and feel fulfilled by the service we provide… service in every sense of the word. Families never forget—nor do we.

Chaplains. No hospice team is complete without its chaplains. They are worth their weight in gold! All hospice chaplains are graduates of special chaplaincy programs, and most are non-denominational in their services. The two chaplains who work with the hospice I serve, for example, can give Catholic communion, but they can also offer prayer and support for those of every other denomination, as well as for agnostics, atheists, and any others whose spirituality falls "outside the lines."

It has been my experience that no matter what faith, if any, a person follows, the approach of death prompts some kind of re-evaluation. Sometimes the patient reconnects to an earlier faith; other times, they find a new way of understanding spirituality entirely. Either way, they almost always feel the need to connect with the divine in some way during this journey. For this reason, I encourage both patients and families to avail themselves of chaplaincy services. Even a patient who does not believe in a "God" can find great comfort in the support of these professionals who are comfortable with, and versed in, spiritual questions of all kinds.

I recently admitted to our service a patient who was dying in a nursing home. Ilene's two daughters and one granddaughter were holding a twenty-four-hour a day vigil to be sure she would not die alone. When I asked if they wanted our chaplain, their first response was to decline. But as we spoke further just before my departure, they agreed to a visit.

I left a message for our chaplain that same day, as I was not sure the patient would live through the night. As it turned out, she did not get my message until much later that night. She visited the first thing in the morning, arriving just before the patient took her final breath. The family deeply appreciated her presence there, and her prayer that their loved one would be carried sweetly to her eternal home.

Hospice volunteers. The last but certainly not least team member is the hospice volunteer. Volunteers are truly the backbone of hospice. In fact, when I first started doing hospice work in 1979, virtually all hospice workers were volunteers. The hospice's executive director, medical director, and the director of clinical nursing were among the only exceptions. Today, most hospices have considerable paid and professional staff. Yet volunteers are still essential. In fact, according to the Hospice Federation, volunteer hours must make up a minimum of five percent of all hospice hours.

Hospice volunteers are mostly, though not always, people who have experienced hospice care during the death of a family member or friend, and then want to give back to this resource that has given their loved one(s) so much. This deeply personal—even passionate—element of their work is one of the things that makes them so valuable to the hospice team. They really serve from the heart.

Though the exact training differs, volunteers at every hospice receive detailed training in ethics, confidentiality, patient support, and other key issues. Obviously, they are not permitted to offer hands-on care of the type that doctors, nurses, or aides provide. Yet what they do is vital. They help with practical necessities like providing transportation, doing errands, and letting families take a much needed break. It is often difficult for people to talk about death and emotions with those around them, so sometimes it is a hospice volunteer that a patient or family confides in, rather than another family member or a more "official" care provider. In hospices that have an actual hospice house, volunteers may staff the kitchen or entrance desk, read to patients, play soft music in the common areas, and/or help with some of the myriad practical tasks involved in running such a facility.

Whenever possible, our hospice tries to match volunteers with families that have similar backgrounds, experiences, or interests. For instance, we might try to connect a volunteer with military experience with a patient who is also a veteran. We are also aware of the many special skills our volunteers may bring to the table, from Reiki training to skills in music or art therapy. Theresa's therapeutic work with puppets, which I discussed earlier in this book, is a perfect example. Hospice budgets rarely have funds for such specialized, "non-essential" help. Yet Theresa's puppets—and Theresa herself—were hugely helpful to Lina and to her family as well. How fortunate we are to be able to count on such loving and talented volunteer support.

As evidence of how generous and thoughtful volunteers' support for families can be, I might add that our volunteers often remain friends with the families they have assisted for years after the patient's death. This can also be true of nurses and aides, of course. Yet the truth is that for those of us that do our hospice work through paid full-time jobs, schedules can simply be too busy to allow us to keep in touch as much as we might like to.

Contracted professionals. To supplement the work of the core hospice team, consultants may be contracted to provide special services. Nutritionists, wound care specialists, physical therapists, occupational therapists, and speech pathologists can all offer crucial help to patients and families. Some individuals require no such services, while others need one or several specialists. Having these experts available as needed is a crucial part of good hospice care.

Why Hospice?

I was pleased but surprised to hear from my old friend Elizabeth Weber one day in September 2008. I had met Elizabeth at college, but she now lived a thousand or so miles away from me and we had lost touch for over ten years. She said she was not exactly sure why she was calling me, but she had had a strong impulse to do so. I had recently begun this book, so it made perfect sense to me! Matter of factly, I told her that I thought she had something I needed for my book. I guess I shouldn't have been surprised when she replied, "Well, my husband did die eight months ago, and we were without friends or family close by at the time. We didn't sign on at first, but hospice was my saving grace." As a way to introduce the question of "why hospice?" in general terms, I want to share her story.

Beth is a very spiritual person and a woman of depth and eloquence. Over the four weeks following her first phone call, we had long weekly talks in which she shared her story with me. Robert had been twenty-five years older than she. Over the course of their ten year marriage he had been her soul mate. Her description of their relationship and his final days was tender and soulful.

When Elizabeth's husband's cancer was diagnosed, Elizabeth said "yes" to chemotherapy because she didn't want her husband to think that she had given up on him. The treatment protocol was presented abruptly, without preparation, and with the comment that if Robert didn't have the treatment, he would be dead in two weeks. The doctor "sprang it on us completely unceremoniously, and put it all on me," Elizabeth told me. No social worker or other support staffer was present to help them process the difficult news or assess their various options. The way it was presented to them, the decision had to be made immediately. Inevitably, they responded more out of shock, guilt and fear than with clarity about their true wishes, feelings, values and intentions.

The treatment of Elizabeth's husband was fairly successful, temporarily shrinking the widespread tumors the disease had caused in the short term. But the chemotherapy was "horrific," Elizabeth commented. "It was like something out of a science fiction movie, with gloves and masks and helmets….so toxic, so violent, so sickening that I don't know how we endured it."

As time passed, Elizabeth became more and more aware that this kind of treatment felt wrong to both of them, and also that the decision to undergo it had been done hastily, without either complete honesty or a review of the options. Weeks after the chemotherapy, Elizabeth and her husband came clean with each other about their feelings. Neither had wanted this difficult and debilitating treatment; both had agreed to it only for the other. In my experience, this is not unusual. Many people agree to treatments they fear out of concern for their loved ones and/or fear that if they do nothing, death will be unbearably hard.

Happily, Elizabeth *did* contact hospice after this time. Her first introduction to hospice was similar to the one I use with my new patients. The professional who handled her informational visit told her that hospice did not mean that this was the end and that miracles do happen. Yet as the days passed, Elizabeth also found that hospice gave her permission to accept that her husband was dying and give him the space to let go. Her only regret, she told me, was that she had not called hospice in earlier.

The day Elizabeth's husband died, she was playing a video of him singing the Hawaiian wedding song at his son's wedding. It meant the world to Elizabeth that the hospice home health aide who was bathing him at the time watched the video with her, appreciating Robert not just as that thing called a "patient" but as a human being who had been full of vitality and love. In hospice it is often the small moments that matter most, and so it was that day. Elizabeth will remember those moments forever—and so, most probably, will the home health aide.

Elizabeth's husband died only a few hours later. She was curled up beside him in his bed, talking to him about what a wonderful husband he had been and how much she loved him. She had the time to reassure him that she would be okay after his passing, that he had her "permission" to go—a very important gift loved ones can give hospice patients—and that she would continue to love him until they were reunited. His death was beautiful and peaceful. Painful as the loss was, Elizabeth told me, his serene and dignified passing and the final times they spent together are memories she would not part with.

Elizabeth is now writing her own book. I am pleased to know that our conversations helped inspire it, and honored to be able to share her story here as well. Being able to tell your own story—as many times as it takes—is a crucial part of the grieving process. In addition to helping her heal, Elizabeth's book will surely be a work of art, and I hope you'll look out for it!

Whether or not it was the right choice, Elizabeth and her husband did get some medical benefit from the chemotherapy, and they signed up with hospice early enough to improve the quality of Robert's last days significantly.

Nancy, whom I met serendipitously in the parking lot of the Omega Institute, was not so lucky on either count. Nancy's husband Fred was only forty-eight at the time he was diagnosed with colon cancer. Their doctor prescribed a variety of very aggressive, invasive treatments. The chances that these treatments would work, the side effects they would have, Fred's wishes, and even the possibility of his death were never discussed, nor was the option for hospice presented to them.

The treatments Fred underwent were unsuccessful, and his disease progressed rapidly. There was no time or strength for even a brief conversation about her husband's life, its meaning, his hopes for his legacy, or any of the other topics that can give both the patient and his loved ones a sense of peacefulness and completion. In fact, until an Intensive Care Unit nurse pulled Nancy aside and told her that her husband was dying, she had no idea that death was so imminent.

Nancy's husband died in the ICU, his mouth full of sores, entangled in a web of wires and tubes.

Nancy and her husband were effectively denied the chance for emotional closure and a serene death. Similarly, had Elizabeth and her husband been offered the option of hospice, they would have had access to a social worker, who would have helped support them in making the right decisions. The issues of quality of life, not just length of life, would have been affirmed and explored. They would have been encouraged to take at least a bit of time to talk with each other, to come clean about their feelings, to ask questions, and to evaluate their options. Whatever their choices were, Elizabeth and her husband would have been able to make those choices based on better information, both objective and subjective.

As this suggests, there is a question of "when hospice" as well as "why" hospice. I'll speak about that more in the next chapter, but for now, let me just emphasize that far from being a doom-filled option to be staved off to the last moment, I believe that hospice can provide much more benefit when signed on—or at least discussed—at the time of diagnosis, rather than later on. Relatively few medical doctors are willing or able to deal with the complex emotions that arise when someone is given a terminal diagnosis. All too often, the news is broken to the patient abruptly, with no discussion of their options, and without adequate support in the form of family members or friends around them. In an ideal world, I believe that the option of hospice should be presented at the same time a terminal diagnosis is given, and that no such diagnosis would be offered without a family member and a social worker present to help them process the news.

I don't want to suggest that hospice is some perfect panacea that makes death simple or easy. Nor do I want to imply that fighting a terminal diagnosis or undergoing radical treatment is always wrong. There are patients and families who are ready and willing to battle even an apparently terminal disease and, as I always say, miracles do happen. Finally, though the doctors in both of the stories I have just discussed presented heroic intervention as the only option, this is not always the case. Thankfully, albeit slowly, more and more doctors today are having the courage to resist this approach.

My friend and editor Suzanne speaks of the oncologist who gave her mother her terminal diagnosis with gratitude, for example. "She simply sat and held our hands as she discussed the news," Suzanne says. "She looked into our eyes, and we felt her respect and affection. She told us our options, including the possibility for treatment, but she did not *push* treatment in any way. In fact, in response to Dad's questions she honestly shared her belief that it was not the right route in Mom's situation, and encouraged us to talk and reflect." This doctor recommended hospice and made the first call to them from her office, allowing the family to have their informational visit the next day. Suzanne's mother died less than two weeks later, peacefully and with her family around her.

With all that said, "why hospice?" On its simplest level, that answer is that caring for a seriously ill or dying person twenty-four hours a day is extremely challenging to do without caring, comprehensive, and knowledgeable professional support—and hospice is really the only source for such support in our culture.

The following are some of the most obvious challenges a patient and his or her family face if they try to "go it alone" in the face of a terminal diagnosis. I want to acknowledge before I begin this list that hospice does not swoop in like a team of superheroes and solve all of these problems for patients and their families! Virtually none of these challenges *disappear* entirely once hospice is called in…but with its support, they become infinitely more manageable.

Availability of caregivers. While some individuals can take care of themselves effectively through much of their own final journey, this is not true of every patient. When a patient is incapacitated or immobilized, arranging for sufficient care can be very difficult. Paid non-hospice providers can be staggeringly expensive, may or may not be covered by insurance, and can be difficult to coordinate. When it comes to the care the family itself can provide, there are many challenges as well.

We all know that it is no longer the norm for families to live closely together in a single community, or for communities themselves to be cohesive and tightly interconnected groups. Today's families may be scattered all over the country, or even around the world. All of the adults may have demanding jobs and responsibilities of their own—responsibilities they can rarely drop entirely even to help a terminally ill loved one. Close friends may also live far afield or have their own personal and professional obligations, and the patient may or may not have a local church, or other community whose members can pitch in. While they do not replace non-professional caregiving, hospice nurses, social workers, Chaplains, aides, and volunteers can help ensure that crucial needs are met no matter what.

Pain and symptom management. Fear of pain and suffering is present in almost every patient and family facing a final illness. As I've discussed earlier in this book, non-hospice medical practices are rarely either equipped or willing to reassure them. Heroic interventions remain the norm, emotional support is often nonexistent, practitioners may or may not be experienced with the particular processes of dying itself, and effective pain management may be compromised by restrictions designed to prevent addictions and dependencies—issues that are certainly valid in general but have little relevance for a dying patient. In contrast, hospice medical staffs have specific expertise in the issues of terminal care and the freedom to use all available resources to support quality of life for the patient.

Location. In my 35 years of nursing experience I have heard literally hundreds of patients say "I just want to go home" or "I want to die at home." For many of the reasons discussed in this chapter, this simply may not be possible without hospice. Instead, patients are consigned to hospitals or nursing homes and the various unnecessary treatments, interruptions to privacy, and discomforts these facilities may involve. Hospice takes for granted that a patient who desires to do so has the right to die at home if at all possible, and does everything feasible to make that desire a reality.

Emotional intensity. When people are given a terminal diagnosis, they and those closest to them must often make very difficult and painful decisions. What if any further tests and treatments should be done? What should be done when Daughter A thinks that Dad's medical intervention should be continued but Daughter B does not? Can Mom die at home or must she be moved to a nursing facility for adequate care? It's likely that few of them will have made such decisions before. The many ramifications make these choices extremely difficult to make, especially at a time when everyone may be struggling to deal with scary diagnoses or prognoses. This is one of the aspects of care in which hospice social workers are so valuable. Specifically trained in problem and conflict resolution (among other skills) and with significant experience in such situations, they can help a family make painful decisions effectively and comfortably.

Family dynamics. Even family members having equally good intentions can hold dramatically contrasting views on the patient's treatment and care. And in some cases, everyone's intentions are not the best! As though the decisions to be made and care to be given are not complicated enough, unresolved conflicts from years or even decades before may arise again in the face of these differences, not only erupting but intensifying. I have literally never attended a case where there was not some kind of complicated dynamic in a patient's family. In this respect it is important to point out that non-hospice medical professionals rarely if ever help with family needs or issues. In contrast, the entire hospice team is trained to help support the family. In addition to the actual expertise these hospice staffers provide, sometimes just the presence of an "outsider" can soothe tensions or mediate conflict.

Timeframe unpredictability. Though we as professionals can often estimate (or intuit) the timing of someone's passing in a general way, no one can predict with true accuracy exactly what will happen, or when. This adds a tremendous extra challenge for family caregivers trying to schedule their efforts. No sooner has a rotation of visits or chores been worked out than the situation changes. In one family, the patient may survive far longer than expected. In another, he or she may pass much more quickly. In still another, the kind of care needed may change dramatically from one day to the next as the patient's symptoms, mobility, or comfort level changes. Interdisciplinary and constantly in touch with each other, the hospice team is designed specifically to be able to respond to such changes quickly and provide a continuity of care no matter what transpires.

Varied, heavy, and sometimes specialized workload. Those caring for a dying loved one must cope with a myriad of jobs. Doing laundry, buying groceries, preparing and serving food, giving and refilling medication, keeping a patient who may be weak or immobile clean and comfortable, alerting family and friends to developments, scheduling visits, answering the phone and email, picking friends or family members up at the airport, paying monthly bills for a patient who may no longer be able to do so him- or herself…the list of tasks involved goes on, and on, and on. Family caregivers may never have handled some, or even any, of these tasks before. Who other than a nurse or aide, for example, has training in how to make a bed with a person in it? Bathe a person who cannot move? Give medications to a drowsy person? Hospice helps to provide training in such tasks, as well as to step in to do some of the most difficult and/or important of them.

Rest and respite. Burnout, depression, and "simple" exhaustion are risks for all of those whose family member is dying, particularly when the process is slow or drawn out. Family caregivers must balance the patient's needs with the necessity of keeping up their own physical and emotional strength. Good sleep may or may not be possible for them if the patient is awake or needs care at night. There may not be enough help to allow them to take a real break, handle their own life issues fully, or do what is needed to maintain their own health in the face of a potentially long-term and painful process. As a result, the longer a patient's final journey goes on the more exhausted and stressed his or her caregiving loved ones may be. Hospice staff has a lot of experience in helping family caregivers deal with these realities; realities we encounter every day. The suggestions, strategies, resources and hands-on help we can provide can make all the difference in getting the family through this difficult journey "in one piece."

Hospice will typically pay for a respite service for a specified number of days. Designed to help the family member who needs a break from caregiving or has obligations elsewhere, this allows the patient to be cared for at the local nursing home of the family's choice. The patient receives their medications, meals, bed, and round the clock nursing care, while the family member can take care of themselves without guilt or worry. Not many families take advantage of this service, but it is a very helpful option.

Access to information and resources. Unless they happen to have had another seriously ill friend or family member in the same community, family caregivers typically do not know what local or regional support resources are available, how best to access them, what they cost, which are the best for their particular situation, and so on. As a result, they may feel confused or unable to help with their loved one's issues, and/or find themselves reinventing the wheel just to get basic assistance. Hospice services avoid this by linking each patient not only to its own care but also to information about other resources that may be available in their situation or community. To name just a few examples, hospice staff will know about support groups for patients and families with cancer, heart disease, Parkinson's disease, terminal illness generally, and so on…"meals on wheels" programs…and other local resources that can make a huge difference.

Bereavement counseling and care. Since feelings of guilt, anger, and other emotions are a normal part of grieving, emotional and psychological support can be crucial as a family tries to heal and move on after a death. I have heard from a number of patient families that they have difficulty getting bereavement counseling if their loved one was not signed up with hospice. (In other communities, hospice-sponsored groups, at the very least, are open to all, whether or not their loved one died under hospice care.) Understanding that it serves families as well as patients themselves, after a patient dies, hospice provides follow-up as part of its services. Individual counseling, support groups, newsletters, and other publications may be available, and most hospices also do regular memorial services or other special commemorations as well.

Cost. Issues of medical cost and insurance coverage are too complex and changeable for me to treat either accurately or fully here, and I make no claim to be an expert on the specifics of these matters. Suffice it to say that almost always, signing on with hospice helps reduce the cost of care for a dying patient. Though some restrictions exist, hospice is a medical benefit covered by Medicare, Medicaid, and many if not most private insurers. On the rare occasions where hospice care must be paid for from the family's own pocket, people are often surprised by how affordable it is. At the time and place I am writing this, private payment is less than $150 per day. Because this covers *everything*—the entire spectrum of hospice services from equipment, medications and supplies to medical, nursing, aid, social worker and other visits—it is actually much more affordable than routine medical treatment. In addition, the hospice intake department, which works with insurance and insurance providers every day, is there to help coordinate. As a result, the family no longer has to figure out complicated coverages or deal with a mountain of paperwork on their own—a true relief at a time when they are already dealing with overwhelming challenges.

With all of this down in black and white, it's obvious why it is so hard for families to care for a dying loved one on their own…and how valuable the support of hospice can be. Hence the answer to "why hospice." The support that hospice provides is not only the hands-on care that is the most obvious part of its services—care that can give a dying person the most comfortable and dignified end of life possible. It is also the instruction on how to do crucial tasks, the help finding crucial resources, the emotional support not just for patients themselves but also families. The care offered not just before but also after the patient has died makes hospice such a powerful force, not only in people's dying journeys but also in the lives of these patients, their families and their communities.

Where and When Hospice?

The "where" in hospice varies from hospice program to hospice program. Though they all work according to the same mission and principles, hospice structures differ widely. Most hospices are not-for-profit, for example, while others are for-profit entities; some are very large, and some smaller; some are part of wide networks, some less widely affiliated. All of these variables may affect how and where a hospice works. Sadly, insurance coverage may also play a role in determining both how and where hospice care is provided.

Some hospices maintain a hospice house with some number of inpatient beds in addition to providing outpatient care. These facilities, which are slowly growing in number, offer a middle ground between home and hospital. They provide the family with caregiving support around the clock, allowing them just to be family members again, rather than serving as primary caregivers. At the same time, the practices and, usually, settings of hospice houses are designed to be as residential in feeling as possible.

These facilities are typically small, offering only a few beds. It's likely that the great majority of patients served even by a hospice with such a facility are not treated there, but rather in their own homes. Certainly, excellent hospice care can be provided without an in-patient facility, as is the norm in hospice. Still, hospice houses offer invaluable help for patients who need it most. Happily, their cost is often covered by Medicare as part of hospice service. Private insurance companies may or may not cover them as well.

A colleague of mine told me about her family's experience with a hospice house in Florida. Her mother, Maddie, had been under hospice care at home. "I had been providing round the clock care for Mom but she had now slipped into unconsciousness. Keeping her clean and giving her proper care was becoming very difficult, even with the help of hospice nurses and aides. Dad felt that Mom would have hated having her daughter drained and exhausted in this way!" Eileen's father called their hospice doctor. A bed at the hospice house had just opened up and they moved her mother there by ambulance that same day. Eileen says that "as we walked through doors my father said that it was so beautiful and serene that he wished Mom could see it. She would have loved the soft colors, the flowers, the little playroom designed specifically for children (both child patients and children of visiting families) and the quiet comfort."

Once Eileen's mother was settled in, the family had time to look around her new "residence." Except for the hospital bed and handicapped-access bathroom, little in the setting looked like a medical facility. There was a small library room with books, a garden outside where families could sit or walk, the children's playroom, and clusters of chairs and loveseats where families could gather and speak outside of their loved one's room. A kitchen had coffee, tea, water and small snacks available at all times, and a chair in the room converted to a bed so that family members could stay overnight if they wished. There was no limit to how many could visit or when and plenty of room for the whole group to gather in the room.

"Mom was in her final days by this time. Her temperature had risen, and the nurses showed us how to use washcloths to cool her. They taught us some basic aromatherapy with some oils that have a soothing effect. They checked on her periodically and were there to answer any questions we had, but aside from that our family was never interrupted," Eileen commented. Her mother's room quickly became a home away from home with family members coming in and out, bringing over her favorite blanket, sharing a cup of tea together, and sitting by her mother's bed. Eileen's father in particular felt calmer knowing that his wife would be loved and cared for without having to place unfair demands on their daughter.

It was Eileen's turn to stay with her mother the night before she died. She remembers how quiet the hospice house was and the sound of crickets, birds, and the rain on the many plants in the garden outside—the same sounds they would have heard at home. She sat with her mother and spoke to her, knowing that she needed to speak her heart and sensing that her mom could at least "feel" the love in her voice even though she was not conscious. Eileen spoke of her memories of how wonderful her mother had been, how much she had learned from her, and how much she would miss her. Before she went to sleep, she also reassured her that she would take care of her dad and that it was also okay for her mother to pass on, even explaining to her that she would be honored to be there at that moment, it was okay for Maddie to go while Eileen slept if that was what she wanted.

"Knowing that others were checking on Mom, I fell into my first deep sleep in weeks. The nurses woke me at six a.m., telling me they thought the time was near. Sure enough, less than a half hour later, Mom died in my arms," Eileen told me. She added that she felt the peacefulness, the energy, and the release of that moment through her whole body. She called the family and they had time together around her mom's bed before the various arrangements were made...there was no rush or intrusion and again, it was much like being at home. She commented that she will be grateful to hospice for the rest of her life for giving her mom a way to stay at home as long as possible, then to die in a place that functioned like home even when she could not *literally* be 'at home.'"

Some hospices also have arrangements with local hospitals to give hospice training and/or care within their walls, either in regular patient rooms or in special wings. This means that a patient can be signed on to hospice service even if they cannot be released from hospital confines. As a result, they and their families can benefit from some of the special social worker support, counseling, chaplaincy help, privacy, elimination of constant interruptions and invasive treatments, and other benefits of hospice. This option is not available in all hospitals, but I hope that it is one that will be added to many more as the years progress.

The hospice I work for does not provide patient care "in house" or in the hospital, except for the acute-care benefit limited to symptom management on the rare occasions it cannot be handled at home. Instead, we provide its services in patient homes, nursing homes, assisted living facilities and Veterans Administration hospitals. As I noted above, our goal is to help the patient die at home if this is possible, given that most of them express the wish to do so. If that is not possible—for example, if a patient's situation requires a nursing home—we work to provide the best quality of life with the least invasive interventions.

Such interventions are not always possible to avoid in nursing homes and other such locations if the patient's wishes are not clear and hospice has not been called in. These facilities and their doctors need to protect themselves from liability by making every effort to sustain patients' lives. This may mean repeated resuscitations or frequent trips from a nursing home to the hospital even when they are debilitating, distressing, or ineffective in any long-term way. I can't urge families enough to have a conversation with their loved one to determine his or her true wishes, then to make those wishes clear and known as soon as possible. Similarly, I encourage everyone to share their own desires about end-of-life issues by creating the necessary legal documents, as well as just talking honestly to family and close friends.

That said, most nursing homes actually welcome hospice involvement in cases where a patient is diagnosed with a life-threatening illness. The array of extra services hospice can provide helps to support the patient and family, and takes some pressure off the always-strained nursing home staff.

Let me turn to the final question, "*when* hospice?"

Hospice can be called in for a consultation by any one, at any time. No doctor is needed to make that call or arrange for the first visit. This meeting is considered an informational visit only. It is free, and it involves no pressure to make a decision, much less to "sign up." Nor, as I have said before, is it intended in any way to suggest that there has been some kind of irrevocable death sentence. Instead, its purpose is to provide information, options, and clarity, allowing the patient and/or family to make the best possible choices in the face of painful realities.

Sometimes this meeting is held very early on, and we at hospice do not hear back from the patient for a while. Other times, a patient is signed on to hospice service that very day. A doctor's order is required to sign a patient on to hospice, since certain medical criteria must be met in order for a patient to be signed on. Again, a patient cannot typically be referred to hospice unless a doctor estimates that if the individual's present condition progresses at its normal anticipated rate, the patient will have six months or less to live. All of those who work for and with hospice, however, understand just how many guesses this assessment involves. In the words of the popular phrase, we always expect the best but prepare for the worst.

Elizabeth's story, which I have shared previously, illustrates how difficult it can be for a patient to process the news that their illness is untreatable when no options are discussed, and if no one who is trained to help process the resulting emotions is present. Sadly, my own personal life includes an even more extreme example of this problem. My sister-in-law was diagnosed with cancer of the thymus at the age of only 49, at a time when her two children were still young. She was in the hospital at the time the news that her illness could not be treated was given to her. Her husband had just stepped out when a hospitalist came into her room, abruptly blurted out the news, and just as abruptly left. She was left alone in a state of shock, disbelief, and fear, and as she told me later, she was naturally unable to remember half of what had been said to her.

I have heard many such stories—even when they don't involve someone near and dear to me—they always leave me stunned and furious. It shocks me that we, in the 21st century, still handle one of the most difficult situations any human being can face in such a cold and barbaric manner. In the words of the Hippocratic Oath, our job as medical professionals is to "first, do no harm." There is no doubt in my mind that telling a patient that their death is near in a way that provides no clarity about their choices, no support for their emotions, and no chance to get their many questions answered with compassion *is* harmful….and can cause the patient and family to make decisions that do not feel right, as Elizabeth and her husband did at first.

I truly believe all patients should have the right to have one or more close family members or friends present at the time a terminal diagnosis is given. Equally important, unless the doctor in question is both trained in and comfortable with giving such diagnoses compassionately and discuss the patient's option, I believe they have the right to have a social worker present to help them process the devastating news, understand their options, and ensure that all of their questions get answered. Whether or not they choose hospice does not matter as much as ensuring that they are given the choice and supported throughout their decision-making process.

Suzanne's story, some of which I shared earlier, illustrates what happens when hospice is called in right at the time a patient is first given a diagnosis that makes them eligible. The oncologist who treated Suzanne's mom was unusual in that she was comfortable with, and skilled in, delivering this kind of news. "She held our hands, sat with us as we absorbed it, and gently talked with us about the limited options we had. It was obvious throughout how much she cared about my parents—she treated both of them. I never for one moment felt that she was rushing or pushing us," Suzanne told me. "I know from hearing friends' stories how rare that is."

Because hospice was called in immediately, the family had support right from the start. Suzanne said that it was "amazing. Mom had been quite ill for months and we mostly had been struggling to figure everything out on our own…and now, suddenly, we had this whole caring, expert team behind us. I can't say enough about how valuable their support was. Facing that Mom's death was likely very imminent was such a blow to everyone, especially my dad. Our whole life changed in an instant. To be able to ask all of our questions and get them answered by caring nurses, a doctor specializing in exactly the situation Mom faced, and the counselor who visited probably saved our sanity."

The hospice team who served Suzanne's mother coordinated all of the elements that the family had struggled to handle alone. Prescriptions were written by the hospice doctor based on family calls or nurses' input, filled at a single pharmacy, and delivered to the home. Aides came to help with bathing, nurses visited regularly, oxygen and a hospital bed were ordered and rapidly delivered when they became needed, and the counselor and social worker were available for visits to help with the family's emotional challenges. Someone was on call around the clock to respond if problems with pain and so on arose. "The more I hear others' stories, the more grateful I am for the courage and wisdom Mom's doctor showed in suggesting that we call in hospice immediately," Suzanne told me. "I can't imagine what it would have been like to have to fight against invasive treatments or to struggle with her diagnosis and its consequences alone. Thanks to that doctor, Mom had the kind of death she wanted—one that was consistent with her values and wishes and with the feelings of the rest of the family as well."

Given the logistical and emotional support it can provide, I would always urge patients and families to call hospice earlier rather than later to schedule the informational meeting. Frightening as it can feel to acknowledge that death may be imminent, this visit will arm everyone involved with the best possible information in the most supportive manner, and allow both the patient and the family to live in alignment with their preferences and values right up to the last.

Hospice and Bereavement

When most people think about bereavement, they think about the period that follows a death. In truth, the long process of grieving has usually begun well before the death. Before hospice is called in, most patients and their loved ones have already struggled with a serious illness and heard the frightening news that their condition is no longer treatable. The shock, denial, anger, and other emotions that arise are complex and painful. One of hospice's most valuable benefits is the way it supports patients and families as they take this long and complicated journey. Because our social workers and bereavement counselors are so attuned to the issues that arise along the way, they can validate feelings, offer support, encourage dialogue, and help people on their path through grief. It is not an exaggeration to say that the work they do is as healing as that of any of the medical or clinical staff. And sometimes its most valuable component is simply creating a safe space for people to express their feelings and reflect on their lives.

When one of their family members is dying, families often experience emotions that feel unloving or shameful to them. Wanting some time to themselves or experiencing resentment for the hard work of care feels selfish when their loved one is near death; wanting their loved one to die in order to relieve suffering induces even more guilt. I have been in that place more than once with my own personal experiences of loss. When my sister-in-law was dying, I remember just wanting it to be over—not just for her sake, but for my own. It felt like the longest seven months of my life. I got to experience firsthand the many conflicting feelings hospice patients and their families undergo, and my longtime hospice experience did not make its challenges significantly easier.

As I mention briefly earlier in this book, loss and grief generally heighten family dysfunction. Everyone involved experiences the five stages of grief that Elizabeth Kübler-Ross identified: shock, anger, denial, bargaining and acceptance. But as she also explains, the stages are not fixed or formulaic. Family members do not experience the stages in the same order or at the same time, nor react to them in the same ways. The fact that there are many important decisions to be made when a family member is dying only heightens the tensions and drama. Our job in hospice is to offer support and guidance, holding the space for them to find peace and balance, whatever that might look like for each family member and whenever healing occurs.

For those left behind after a loved one's death, full recovery from grief is a long and unpredictable process. (In truth, I am not sure anyone ever truly "recovers" from a loss, but they do learn to readjust and move on.) For this reason, the work of hospice does not stop when a patient dies. We continue to offer a variety of sources of support. It is not unusual for one or more of the hospice team to attend the funeral or memorial service of a patient they have grown close to. We send a sympathy card to the family within the first week, and our bereavement coordinator or volunteer call the family during the second week. The family is offered a follow-up bereavement visit if they have a need for it, and everyone is encouraged to attend one of our ongoing grief groups as often and for as long as they like. Though every hospice has slightly different practices, almost all send some combination of newsletters, helpful literature, and even a personal note during the first year of bereavement.

In addition, families are invited to call hospice as often as they need to during that first year. Just being reassured that what they are feeling is normal and that they are not going crazy can be a tremendous relief. The journey of grief is often an isolating one in our culture. The bereaved may be avoided by friends who don't know what to say, and their sadness can begin to feel like a brand that sets them apart from "normal life." My dear friend and the editor of this book, Suzanne Fox, called this "wearing the D" in one of the eloquent small books she created in the wake of her parents' deaths. As she says, the "D" seems to stand for death, distance, despair, and even the disappearance of the identity the bereaved person used to have. Yet in the long run it also stands for devotion, depth, and determination that come with healing.

Like many others, my hospice offers two memorial services each year to allow families to gather with others who have lost loved ones during the same period, as well as with members of the hospice team. These services are always moving in the way they honor not only those who have died, but also the loved ones who remember them. In a way, they are yet another reflection of the comment those of us in hospice work so often make, that hospice is not just about death but about life.

Miracles Do Happen

According to Bette Kravetz, one of my dearest friends, the number eighteen is the Hebrew number for a blessed life. To make this final, eighteenth chapter worthy of its sacred number, I have chosen to share one of the real-life stories of hospice that ranks high on my experiences of miracles.

Linda has been a hospice nurse with our agency for over fifteen years. In 1987, when her sons were only seven and nine years old, a hairdresser had noticed a dark, flat, symmetrical mole on her neck and advised Linda to get it checked. Linda finally agreed, but the doctor who looked at it said it was nothing to worry about. Still, the hairdresser would not let up. "I finally realized that I would either need to get a new doctor, or get a new hairdresser—so I chose to change doctors," Linda told me. The new doctor diagnosed the mole as melanoma. "It was as though my whole field of vision tunneled. I couldn't hear or see anything else after hearing the word 'melanoma.'"

Linda was referred to an oncologist who was able to remove the growth without extensive surgery. It remained quiet for many years. During this time she entered hospice nursing. Linda tells me that she did so with the mindset that "if I work in this field, it won't happen to me."

Fifteen years after its first appearance, Linda's melanoma returned. This time around, the prognosis was grim. Two extensive surgeries were done and a course of chemotherapy begun. "It left me feeling diseased and contagious," Linda told me, remembering the medical personnel that seemed to go out of their way to avoid touching her. She remembers to this day her gratitude for the student technician who placed a compassionate hand on her shoulder as though affirming their common humanity.

Despite the many strong treatments, Linda's melanoma continued to recur. Linda continued to work as a hospice nurse in the midst of this until her doctor finally said that he had exhausted all of the possible treatment options.

Linda was much loved in our hospice, and this news left all of us grief-stricken. When Linda wanted to say her good-byes we all gathered around her, holding hands and reciting the Lord's Prayer. Our supervisor had made several hundred pins with the initial "L" on them. The entire staff wore the pins for many months. Many of us prayed for her; I remember praying for her every single day for a solid year. In addition, Linda stood up in her church to ask the congregation for its prayers—a courageous act for someone who, like so many of us, is reluctant to burden others and ask for help. To this day she attributes her miracle to the heartfelt prayers of the many willing people around her, along with her own openness to a new treatment opportunity when it arose.

This new modality was available in a few places. Linda was eventually able to be treated at one of these centers. After several months of treatment and much uncertainty, Linda's good health returned. For the past three years she has been cancer-free and able to resume her full-time work as a hospice nurse.

In the course of writing this book, I asked Linda how she felt that this extraordinary experience had affected her life. She replied, quite simply, that "I have learned the importance of staying in the moment, and doing only that which has real value."

"I probably think about my own death several times a day. I don't shy away from these thoughts or from people who have melanoma or other such conditions. I never bring up my own experience with patients, but most of them sense it. I guess I would say that life is good," she concluded. "The good and the bad—it is *all* good."

Ten Common Myths About Grieving

1. Family members and friends are the best source of support for those in grief. In an ideal world, this might be true—but not in the real one. No matter how much they want to, many people find it hard to support a grieving friend or family member well. All too often their own issues, feelings, histories, or temperaments get in the way. They may not be able to ask what the bereaved person needs, resist offering advice that is not useful or well timed, or cope with the emotions that arise.

For this reason, individual counseling, grief groups, and other resources can be hugely helpful. A trained professional can anticipate some of the issues that arise in bereavement situations and is comfortable discussing the full range of feelings that come up without judgment. In a confidential setting and/or among peers they do not know well personally, a grieving person may actually feel more comfortable speaking up, "venting," crying, or acknowledging difficult feelings honestly.

2. Family fights or conflicts mean that the family does not grieve for the dying person. As I have said elsewhere in this book, almost every family has some complicated dynamic or other and the "eruption" of these dynamics often continues even after the loved one has died. Even when they get ugly, these conflicts do not mean that participants in them don't care or are not grieving. In fact, the opposite is often true. Family members may behave badly because they *do* care, because anger or disputes help them shield themselves from their powerlessness and pain in the aftermath of loss.

3. Death and grief need to be hidden from children. This is not true…but even if it were, I don't believe it would be possible! Children are much more intuitive and aware than most of us adults are. Pretending that nothing is wrong when they can see doctors visiting, adults crying, loved ones in pain, equipment being set up, and so on may only make death and loss scarier for them by denying the reality they clearly perceive. The facts of death, dying, loss and healing can and should be communicated in age-appropriate ways. But within that limitation, I always encourage parents to take their cue from the child. Children will set the tone if given the opportunity. They typically only request that information they can handle, and will raise questions or concerns in different ways over time as necessary to help them process. When I am asked if children should attend funerals, I always say "by all means—if the child wants to."

4. Expected deaths are less painful for surviving friends and family. The truth is that death can be profoundly challenging for survivors no matter what the timeframe. Having time to process a diagnosis can allow emotions to be expressed and goodbyes to be said. But watching a loved one refuse to eat, linger for long periods, "waste away," or experience discomfort can be just as painful as having to deal with a sudden death. It is not really helpful to make comparisons or judgments of this kind.

5. The progress of grief can be predicted. Dr. Elisabeth Kübler-Ross, among others, identified emotions and stages of grief….but the timing, sequence, and intensity of these stages is anything but standardized. There is no universal "normal" in this regard, no "right" way to grieve, and no single timeframe in which grieving should be finished. One person may feel a great deal of anger against God, death, or even the deceased loved one who has left them. Another may be conscious of little anger at all. One person may experience lots of feelings right after the death, while another may not fully work through all of the stages of grief for months or even years.

6. Grieving people want you to "help" them. In my experience, the family members and friends who survive the loss of someone significant are often most grateful for a quiet, accepting presence… someone who honors their emotions, respects their choices, listens to their stories, and accepts their pain rather than trying to fix them or the situation.

7. The first days and weeks are the most painful. Sometimes this is true, but sometimes not. Shock may dull the pain in the early days, even when the loss is "expected." Visitors, financial and legal tasks, memorial and funeral events may keep the surviving spouse, parent, or children very busy right after a death, leaving the full grief, sadness, loss and loneliness to be experienced later on. Key dates and anniversaries—holidays, the loved one's birthday, and the date of death, for example—sometimes cause grief that has seemed calmer to arise again.

8. You will upset a bereaved person by mentioning their loved one or their loss. Some grieving people end up being temporarily abandoned by their friends, each of whom feels that it is better to stay away entirely than risk saying the wrong thing! In reality, mentioning the loved one or the loss in some gentle way is rarely a shock or surprise to someone in grief. Instead, it actually invites the grieving person to be "real" with you about their feelings if they wish to do so.

9. Feeling deep grief means that you do not believe in God, have faith, believe in an afterlife, etc. Many people assume that those who have deep spiritual convictions will feel grief less than those who do not. This is a myth. When faced with the passing of a loved one, pain and questioning are natural for those of all beliefs, and no beliefs. Believing that someone has gone "to a better place" does not mean that the one left behind does not miss them deeply on earth, mourn their passing profoundly, and experience challenging pain. This is probably why most of the major religious traditions, even those that believe in a beautiful afterlife, offer nurturing rituals, prayers, and other support systems for those who lose a loved one.

10. The best way to heal is to keep busy. This advice is often given to bereaved people, but is not always the best strategy. There is no single "best way" to heal from loss. Everything to do with death and dying is extremely personal. Each person must and will find the path that works best for them. Urging meaningless busywork or social activities on someone who is grieving can serve to make them feel lazy, guilty, or inadequate rather than soothed or supported. Often when people keep themselves too busy, they are only postponing the grieving process. We call it grief "work" because it IS work. It is important that people allow themselves to feel their pain and sadness, and embrace the fact that their lives have been changed forever. Grief is a long and lonely journey that each person must someday go through....with or without the help of hospice.

In Conclusion

Though I have been involved with hospice for over thirty years now, I have only had the privilege of being present as a patient took his or her last breath on a handful of occasions. I would like to close with one such precious memory.

I was on call when I received a call from Tammy, the daughter of our hospice patient, Mary. Mary was in her mid-forties and suffered from a rare respiratory disease. Her daughter felt very fearful about her mother's impending death; her most troubling fear was that her mother would die gasping for breath. It has been my own experience that patients with lung cancer, COPD, and other respiratory issues usually die quite peacefully, without struggling for air, thanks in part to the morphine they are often on at the end. However, I also sympathize with the fears of those like Tammy, who above all want to ensure that their loved ones are comfortable right to the end.

When Tammy called me, she was panicked. She told me that she thought her mother had died, but she wasn't entirely sure. I had been on this case for many months and was eager to come to her aid even though it was eight p.m. by the time the call came in. The fact that Mary's disease was so rare did make me nervous, I have to admit. Without experience with this particular illness, I could not be sure how her last minutes would play out.

A houseful of friends and family had gathered by the time I arrived. I knew most of them fairly well by this time. Mary was still alive, but her vital signs indicated that her death was near. For some reason I can't entirely explain—perhaps because I have studied reflexology—I felt guided to be at her feet. As I usually do, I encouraged the family to talk about old times and favorite family memories. As I have mentioned previously, hearing is generally accepted to be the last sense that goes as a patient dies. It is my belief that these loving words are heard, or at least felt. I prayed silently for a smooth journey while holding Mary's feet in my hands; grouped around the head of the bed, her family spoke of what a loving mother and woman she had been. I remember her daughter wiping her mother's forehead while whispering in her ear. As we waited there, Mary began to take her final breaths. They were calm, graceful, and even leisurely. Mary took her last breath peacefully, the last noises she heard being sounds of love and appreciation.

When her daughter realized that her mother had died, her relief was palpable. "Look at her!" she said. Her voice was loud with emotion and tears; tears —of joy, of relief, of grief—were streaming down her face. "Look how beautiful and peaceful she looks. There isn't any struggle... she looks so happy!"

I have quoted Carol, our chaplain, before. She often comments that "Every time I am present at the time of a person's last breath, I am in awe...I am in *awe.*" I too was in awe that night. Coupled with the sadness of great loss was the heartfelt celebration that Mary had died so peacefully and that the illness that had troubled her so deeply for so long was now over. It was sacred, sad, and yet also a joyous time. For some reason, I still recall bending over the toddler gate that had been installed—I don't remember whether it was for the benefit of children or pets—and kissing Mary's son, who was lying on the living room floor.

I said my goodbyes to the family with gratitude for the opportunity to experience this extraordinary moment with them. I was reminded yet again of what a gift my patients, their families, and the experiences I share with them are. Naturally, there are moments that are tiring or frustrating, moments when wires cross or schedules fall apart or circumstances are less than ideal. Yet these are far outnumbered by the times that teach me, nurture me, amaze me, inspire me, and fill me with joy. I have said with what may be annoying frequency that ultimately, hospice is not about death but about quality of life. It seems fitting to end this story of my hospice work with the heartfelt acknowledgement that one of the lives whose quality hospice has enhanced the most is undoubtedly my own.

About the Author

Cathy Truehart's training in nursing began in 1971. In 1974, she earned a Diploma in Nursing from Worcester City Hospital School of Nursing in Massachusetts. In 1981, she earned a BSN in Public Health Nursing with a minor in Gerontology from California State University in Cotati, California, where she also did a year-long preceptorship with Hospice of Sonoma County. Finally, in 1997 Cathy completed her Masters Degree in counseling psychology at Leslie College in Cambridge, Massachusetts.

Cathy's longstanding interest in holistic health has motivated her to complete a certification program in holistic nursing through Seeds & Bridges; a practitioner degree in Neuro-Linguistic Programming; advanced Reiki certification; and a certification in reflexology.

Currently, Cathy is working as a hospice nurse in western Massachusetts and Volunteer and Bereavement Coordinator in Connecticut. She has been married to her husband, Richard Truehart, for thirty years, and is the very proud mother of two beautiful daughters, Crystal Rose and Rachel Rose.

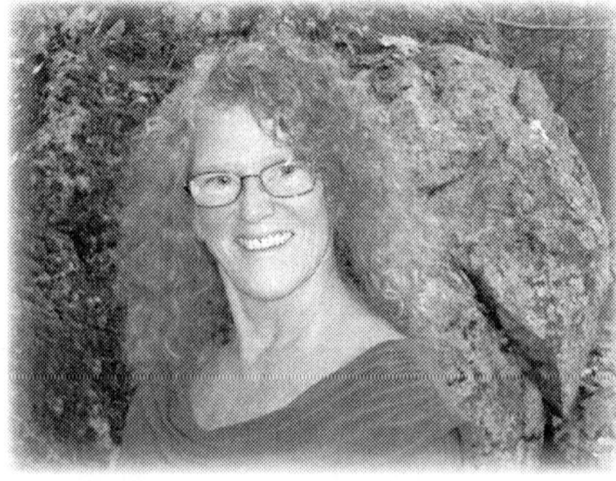

Visit the author's blog at www.miracleofhospice.wordpress.com

Acknowledgements

My first and most grateful acknowledgement is to my husband, Richard, who has been so patient with me and allowed me the time to manifest my dream of writing a book. Richard, I am more grateful than you know. Because of you, I am able to live my life the way I want. God bless you, dear—I love you so very much. Second "in line" for my love and thanks are my daughters, Rachel Rose and Crystal Rose, who are beautiful young women in body, mind, and spirit.

I want to thank my first readers, who gave me such wise, warm feedback on the earlier drafts of this book. Kris Wailgum, Bettie Kravetz, Cheryl Kennedy, Shirley Rogers, Carole Schulte, Faith Sullivan, JoAnn Slosek, Donna Estes, and Philomena Gaida all gave me a way to test out this work on an audience that was honest, insightful, and supportive, and I am very grateful. A special thank you to JoAnn Slosek for the title of this book.

My friend Elsa Weber (also referred to Elizabeth Weber) was a special source of inspiration and support as I wrote this book. I thank her gratefully, and wish her well with her own book.

My great thanks go to my freelance editor, Suzanne Fox, who became a dear friend upon our very first meeting. Her experience not only in books and writing, but also as a person dealing with loss and hospice herself, made her an invaluable voice in this manuscript. Without her, this book would never have materialized. Thank you so very much, Suzanne, for your guidance, your support and your ability to make sense out of my scribbling.

I would also like to thank my colleagues Linda Twyeffort, Madeline LaFlamme, Mary Sheehan and David Rosenberger for sharing their personal stories and expertise; though I have acknowledged Carole Schulte already, she offered great help in this regard as well.

My thanks go as well to my dear friends Donna Egan, Cheryl Kennedy, and Darcy Truehart—both a sister-in-law and a friend—for being such compassionate listeners and supporters of the work I do; to my sister Donna Vaughan for our wonderful writing retreats; and to my mother, Olive Wells, who is my biggest cheerleader and confidante.

Last but very much not least, my heartfelt thanks go to all of my hospice patients and families; past, present, and future. As I said in this book's Dedication, it is my deepest privilege to serve them.

For Further Exploration

There are so many excellent websites, books, and DVDs related to hospice, dying, grief, and caregiving that it is impossible to list even a fraction of available resources. The list that follows is just a very small sampling of my own personal favorites.

Please note that while the information provided here is correct as of the date I am writing, it is of course subject to change over time. No mention of a site or organization here constitutes an endorsement or recommendation; all resources listed are merely a starting point for your own exploration.

Web Sites

Hospice organizations including the National Hospice and Palliative Care Organization (www.nhpco.org) and the Hospice Foundation of America (www.hospicefoundation.org) have rich and helpful web sites. As caregiving becomes more and more a part of American lives, good Internet resources on caregiving have grown as well. A variety of organizations including the National Family Caregivers Association, (www.thefamilycaregiver.org), the National Alliance for Caregiving (www.caregiving.org)and the Family Caregiver Alliance (www.caregiver.org), among others, provide valuable information, education, and advocacy. Family Caregiving 101 (www.familycaregiving101.org) is also helpful in identifying and framing critical questions a caregiver faces.

Books

If multiple editions of a given book exist, I have listed the publisher of the most recent and/or widely available one. Where possible, I have also provided the author's website in the listings below. If no author website is given, one was not available at the time of this writing.

I discussed the pioneering Dr. Elisabeth Kübler-Ross in Chapter 13 of this book. You can find out more about this remarkable woman, her books, and her lasting impact on our culture on the website of the Elisabeth Kübler-Ross Foundation (www.ekrfoundation.org). One of my personal favorites among her work is *The Wheel of Life*. On the subject of dying, I also recommend Ellen Tadd's *Death and Letting Go* (Montague Press; www.ellentadd.com); *The Needs of the Dying: A Guide for Bringing Hope, Comfort and Love to Life's Final Chapter* by David Kessler, who collaborated with Dr. Kübler-Ross on several of her books and worked in hospice for over twenty years (Harper Paperbacks; www.grief.com); and *Final Gifts: Understanding the Special Awareness, Needs, and Communication of the Dying* by Maggie Callanan and Patricia Kelley, which shares the insights on dying gathered from the two authors' long work as hospice nurses (Bantam Books; www.maggiecallanan.com).

Personal favorite books on the subject of complementary medicine include Laura Norman's Feet First: A Guide to Foot Reflexology (Touchstone Books; www.lauranorman.com). Nurses interested in the use of complementary medicine in their professional work may wish to consult Holistic Nursing: A Handbook for Practice by Barbara Dossey, Lynn Keegan, and Cathie Guzzetta (Jones & Bartlett Learning; wwwjblearning.com, www.dosseydossey.com).

On the subject of spirituality, I have learned much from the Course in Miracles (Foundation for Inner Peace; www.acim.org) and from Marianne Williamson, notably her book *Return to Love* (Harper Paperbacks; www.marianne.com), which reflects on the Course in Miracles.

The small books on grief created by my editor on this project, Suzanne Fox, offer lovely support to the newly bereaved. They include *Grief Country* and *Wearing the D* and can be found on Suzanne's website, www.bookstrategy.com.

Memoirs and personal histories enrich our understanding of the different ways loss, healing and grace work in our lives. My list of favorites begins with the extraordinary and healing *A Beautiful Mourning* by my friend Elsa Weber (www.elsaweber.com). Colleagues, friends and patients mention Tim Brookes' *Signs of Life* (Times Books; www.timbrookesinc.com); Judy Collins' *Sanity and Grace* (Tarcher/Penguin; www.judycollins.com); Ann Hood's *Comfort;* (W.W. Norton & Co.;

www.annhood.us); Kay Jamison's *Nothing Was The Same* (Vintage Books); Elizabeth McCracken's *An Exact Replica of a Figment of My Imagination* (Jonathan Cape Books; www.elizabethmccracken.com); Meghan O'Rourke's *The Long Goodbye* (Riverhead Books; www.meghanorourke.net; and Anne Roiphe's *Epilogue: A Memoir* (Harper Books) as moving and helpful. Further exploration will surely yield books which speak to your own situation, needs and values.

Audio and Video

There are so many excellent audio programs, audio downloads, videos and films on the subjects of healing and grief today that as with books, it's impossible to list even a fraction of the available resources. Just a very few of my personal favorites follow. Several of the resources listed under books above are also available in audio CD or download format.

First published in 1999, Gary Zukav's *The Seat of the Soul* is now a classic. It can be purchased in book, CD, or audio download form through www.seatofthesoul.com.

One of my favorite works on complementary healing is available through excellent DVDs as well as in book form. It is Donna Eden's *Energy Medicine,* and it can be purchased in the form of your choice on Donna's website, www.innersource.net.

The Science of Medical Intuition by Caroline Myss and Norm Shealy, MD is just one of Myss's many powerful programs. It is available from www.soundstrue.com, while a variety of Myss's other audio downloads, DVDs, and books are available on her website at www.myss.com.

Angel and Executioner: Grief and the Love of Life is a live recording of Stephen Jenkinson speaking about themes including his belief that "the meaning of the end of your life must be made instead of found." I also highly recommend *Griefwalker,* a film about Jenkinson's extraordinary work with the dying, directed by Tim Wilson and produced by the National Film Board of Canada. Both can be found at www.orphanwisdom.com.

CPSIA information can be obtained at www.ICGtesting.com
Printed in the USA
BVOW010009021012

301852BV00003B/1/P